Ubaldo Leli, MD
Jack Drescher, MD
Editors

M000218045

Transgender Subjectivities: A Clinician's Guide

Transgender Subjectivities: A Clinician's Guide has been co-published simultaneously as *Journal of Gay & Lesbian Psychotherapy*, Volume 8, Numbers 1/2 2004.

*Pre-publication
REVIEWS,
COMMENTARIES,
EVALUATIONS . . .*

"IMPORTANT. . . . IMPRESSIVE. . . . The particular value of this book is its presentation, via personal histories, clinical research, statistical data, and relevant clinical vignettes of the subjective world of individuals occupying that 'intergender' culturally embattled space of transsexuality and transgenderism. INDISPENSABLE for diagnosticians and therapists dealing with gender dysphoria, IMPORTANT for researchers, and A DIRECT SOURCE OF HELP for all individuals suffering from painful uncertainties regarding their sexual identity."

Otto F. Kernberg, MD
*Director
Personality Disorders Institute
Weill Medical College of Cornell University*

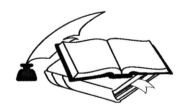

More pre-publication
REVIEWS, COMMENTARIES, EVALUATIONS . . .

"IMPORTANT. . . . AN EXCELLENT COMPILATION. . . . Starts strong with two riveting first-person accounts of transsexualism, one of them on a psychiatrist's transformation from male to female."

Ethel Spector Person, MD
Professor of Clinical Psychiatry
College of Physicians and Surgeons
Columbia University
Author
The Sexual Century

"IN THIS PATHBREAKING WORK, Leli and Drescher have collected valuable clinical papers and personal accounts to provide clinicians with new ideas and a broader understanding of adult gender dysphoric and transgender individuals. Mental health practitioners will find themselves emotionally moved, challenged to rethink assumptions, and opened to provocative questions, as they explore several excellent contributions on the experiences of transgendered individuals."

Eleanor Schuker, MD
Training and Supervising Analyst
Columbia University Center
for Psychoanalytic Training
and Research

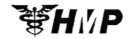

The Haworth Medical Press
An Imprint of The Haworth Press, Inc.

Transgender Subjectivities: A Clinician's Guide

Transgender Subjectivities: A Clinician's Guide has been co-published simultaneously as *Journal of Gay & Lesbian Psychotherapy*, Volume 8, Numbers 1/2 2004.

The *Journal of Gay & Lesbian Psychotherapy* Monographic "Separates"

Below is a list of "separates," which in serials librarianship means a special issue simultaneously published as a special journal issue or double-issue *and* as a "separate" hardbound monograph. (This is a format which we also call a "DocuSerial.")

"Separates" are published because specialized libraries or professionals may wish to purchase a specific thematic issue by itself in a format which can be separately cataloged and shelved, as opposed to purchasing the journal on an on-going basis. Faculty members may also more easily consider a "separate" for classroom adoption.

"Separates" are carefully classified separately with the major book jobbers so that the journal tie-in can be noted on new book order slips to avoid duplicate purchasing.

You may wish to visit Haworth's website at . . .

http://www.HaworthPress.com

. . . to search our online catalog for complete tables of contents of these separates and related publications.

You may also call 1-800-HAWORTH (outside US/Canada: 607-722-5857), or Fax: 1-800-895-0582 (outside US/Canada: 607-771-0012), or e-mail at:

docdelivery@haworthpress.com

Transgender Subjectivities: A Clinician's Guide, edited by Ubaldo Leli, MD, and Jack Drescher, MD (Vol. 8, No. 1/2, 2004). *"INDISPENSABLE for diagnosticians and therapists dealing with gender dysphoria, important for researchers, and a direct source of help for all individuals suffering from painful uncertainties regarding their sexual identity." (Otto F. Kernberg, MD, Director, Personality Disorders Institute, Weill Medical College of Cornell University)*

The Mental Health Professions and Homosexuality: International Perspectives, edited by Vittorio Lingiardi, MD, and Jack Drescher, MD (Vol. 7, No. 1/2, 2003). *"PROVIDES A WORLDWIDE PERSPECTIVE that illuminates the psychiatric, psychoanalytic, and mental health professions' understanding and treatment of both lay and professional sexual minorities." (Bob Barrett, PhD, Professor and Counseling Program Coordinator, University of North Carolina at Charlotte)*

Sexual Conversion Therapy: Ethical, Clinical, and Research Perspectives, edited by Ariel Shidlo, PhD, Michael Schroeder, PsyD, and Jack Drescher, MD (Vol. 5, No. 3/4, 2001)."*THIS IS AN IMPORTANT BOOK. . . . AN INVALUABLE RESOURCES FOR MENTAL HEALTH PROVIDERS AND POLICYMAKERS. This book gives voice to those men and women who have experienced painful, degrading, and unsuccessful conversion therapy and survived. The ethics and misuses of conversion therapy practice are well documented, as are the harmful effects." (Joyce Hunter, DSW, Research Scientist, HIV Center for Clinical & Behavioral Studies, New York State Psychiatric Institute/Columbia University, New York City)*

Gay and Lesbian Parenting, edited by Deborah F. Glazer, PhD, and Jack Drescher, MD (Vol. 4, No. 3/4, 2001). *Richly textured, probing. These papers accomplish a rare feat: they explore in a candid, psychologically sophisticated, yet highly readable fashion how parenthood impacts lesbian and gay identity and how these identities affect the experience of parenting. Wonderfully informative. (Martin Stephen Frommer, PhD, Faculty/Supervisor, The Institute for Contemporary Psychotherapy, New York City).*

Addictions in the Gay and Lesbian Community, edited by Jeffrey R. Guss, MD, and Jack Drescher, MD (Vol. 3, No. 3/4, 2000). *Explores the unique clinical considerations involved in addiction treatment for gay men and lesbians, groups that reportedly use and abuse alcohol and substances at higher rates than the general population.*

Transgender Subjectivities: A Clinician's Guide

Ubaldo Leli, MD
Jack Drescher, MD
Editors

Transgender Subjectivities: A Clinician's Guide has been co-published simultaneously as *Journal of Gay & Lesbian Psychotherapy*, Volume 8, Numbers 1/2 2004.

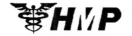

The Haworth Medical Press®
Harrington Park Press®
Imprints of The Haworth Press, Inc.

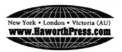

New York • London • Victoria (AU)
www.HaworthPress.com

Published by

The Haworth Medical Press®, 10 Alice Street, Binghamton, NY 13904-1580 USA

The Haworth Medical Press® is an imprint of The Haworth Press, Inc., 10 Alice Street, Binghamton, NY 13904-1580 USA.

Transgender Subjectivities: A Clinician's Guide has been co-published simultaneously as *Journal of Gay & Lesbian Psychotherapy*, Volume 8, Numbers 1/2 2004.

The development, preparation, and publication of this work has been undertaken with great care. However, the publisher, employees, editors, and agents of The Haworth Press and all imprints of The Haworth Press, Inc., including The Haworth Medical Press® and Pharmaceutical Products Press®, are not responsible for any errors contained herein or for consequences that may ensue from use of materials or information contained in this work. Opinions expressed by the author(s) are not necessarily those of The Haworth Press, Inc. With regard to case studies, identities and circumstances of individuals discussed herein have been changed to protect confidentiality. Any resemblance to actual persons, living or dead, is entirely coincidental.

Cover design by Lora L. Wiggins

Library of Congress Cataloging-in-Publication Data

Transgender subjectivities : a clinician's guide / Ubaldo Leli, Jack Drescher, editors.
        p. cm.
        "Co-published simultaneously as Journal of gay & lesbian psychotherapy, volume 8, number 1/2 2004."
        Includes bibliographical references and index.
    ISBN 0-7890-2575-2 (hard cover : alk. paper) – ISBN 0-7890-2576-0 (soft cover : alk. paper)
        1. Transsexualism. 2. Psychotherapy. I. Leli, Ubaldo. II. Drescher, Jack, 1951-
RC560.G45T73 2004
616.89'14'08664–dc22
                                                                                2004009973

Indexing, Abstracting & Website/Internet Coverage

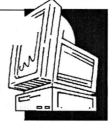

This section provides you with a list of major indexing & abstracting services. That is to say, each service began covering this periodical during the year noted in the right column. Most Websites which are listed below have indicated that they will either post, disseminate, compile, archive, cite or alert their own Website users with research-based content from this work. (This list is as current as the copyright date of this publication.)

Abstracting, Website/Indexing Coverage . . . . Year When Coverage Began

- *Abstracts in Anthropology* 1991
- *Academic Index (on-line)* 1992
- *Academic Search Elite (EBSCO)* 1998
- *Academic Search Premier (EBSCO)* 2001
- *Business Source Corporate: coverage of nearly 3,350 quality magazines and journals; designed to meet the diverse information needs of corporations; EBSCO Publishing <http://www.epnet.com/corporate/bsourcecorp.asp>* 1998
- *Contemporary Women's Issues* 1998
- *e-psyche, LLC <http://www.e-psyche.net>* 2001
- *Expanded Academic ASAP <http://www.galegroup.com>* 1993
- *Expanded Academic ASAP–International <http://www.galegroup.com>* 1993
- *Expanded Academic Index* 1995
- *Family Index Database <http://www.familyscholar.com>* 2003
- *Family Violence & Sexual Assault Bulletin* 1992
- *GenderWatch <http://www.slinfo.com>* 1999
- *GLBT Life, EBSCO Publishing <http://www.epnet.com/academic/glbt.asp>* 2004

(continued)

(continued)

    *Exact start date to come.

*Special Bibliographic Notes related to special journal issues
(separates) and indexing/abstracting:*

- indexing/abstracting services in this list will also cover material in any "separate" that is co-published simultaneously with Haworth's special thematic journal issue or DocuSerial. Indexing/abstracting usually covers material at the article/chapter level.
- monographic co-editions are intended for either non-subscribers or libraries which intend to purchase a second copy for their circulating collections.
- monographic co-editions are reported to all jobbers/wholesalers/approval plans. The source journal is listed as the "series" to assist the prevention of duplicate purchasing in the same manner utilized for books-in-series.
- to facilitate user/access services all indexing/abstracting services are encouraged to utilize the co-indexing entry note indicated at the bottom of the first page of each article/chapter/contribution.
- this is intended to assist a library user of any reference tool (whether print, electronic, online, or CD-ROM) to locate the monographic version if the library has purchased this version but not a subscription to the source journal.
- individual articles/chapters in any Haworth publication are also available through the Haworth Document Delivery Service (HDDS).

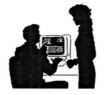

Transgender Subjectivities:
A Clinician's Guide

CONTENTS

ABOUT THE EDITORS

Ubaldo Leli, MD, is a Lecturer in Psychiatry at the Columbia University College of Physician and Surgeons, Clinical Associate in Psychiatry at Weill Cornell Medical College and New York-Presbyterian Hospital, a member of the faculty at the Columbia Center for Psychoanalytic Training and Research, and maintains a full-time private practice in New York City.

Jack Drescher, MD, is a Fellow, Training and Supervising Analyst at the William Alanson White Psychoanalytic Institute and Clinical Assistant Professor of Psychiatry at SUNY-Downstate. He is Past President of the New York County District Branch, American Psychiatric Association and Chair of the Committee on GLB Concerns of the APA. Author of *Psychoanalytic Therapy and the Gay Man* (1998, The Analytic Press) and Editor-in-Chief of the *JGLP*, Dr. Drescher is in private practice in New York City.

Crossing Over:
Introduction

In this special monograph issue of the *Journal of Gay & Lesbian Psychotherapy,* the focus returns once again to the clinical issues and concerns of transgendered individuals. As Aaron (formerly Holly) Devor put it in the *JGLP's* first visit to this subject:

> [B]oth historically and cross-culturally, transgender people have been the most visible minority among people involved in same-sex sexual practices. As such, transgendered people have been emblematic of homosexuality in the minds of most people. Thus, the concerns of gay, lesbian, bisexual [GLB] and queer people are inextricably bound up with those of transgendered people and should be addressed together in LGBT groups. (Devor, 2002, pp. 5-6)

The impetus to publish the papers in this volume–which together offer several snapshots of transgender presentations and subjectivities–reflects a growing awareness of gender non-conformity and gender dysphoria within the mental health community at large. Many mental health practitioners now find themselves challenged by questions raised by transgendered individuals who present for psychotherapeutic treatment, either for a gender issue per se, or for other reasons.

It is no surprise to readers of this journal that many GLB patients, both in the United States and elsewhere, find it difficult to obtain appropriate, respectful treatment from practitioners sensitive to their unique cultural concerns. The situation seems even more bleak for the much smaller group of patients

[Haworth co-indexing entry note]: "Crossing Over: Introduction." Leli, Ubaldo, and Jack Drescher. Co-published simultaneously in *Journal of Gay & Lesbian Psychotherapy* (The Haworth Medical Press, an imprint of The Haworth Press, Inc.) Vol. 8, No. 1/2, 2004, pp. 1-5; and: *Transgender Subjectivities: A Clinician's Guide* (ed: Ubaldo Leli, and Jack Drescher) The Haworth Medical Press, an imprint of The Haworth Press, Inc., 2004, pp. 1-5. Single or multiple copies of this article are available for a fee from The Haworth Document Delivery Service [1-800-HAWORTH, 9:00 a.m. - 5:00 p.m. (EST). E-mail address: docdelivery@haworthpress.com].

http://www.haworthpress.com/web/JGLP
© 2004 by The Haworth Press, Inc. All rights reserved.
Digital Object Identifer: 10.1300/J236v08n01_01

1

with gender dysphoria. Not only does the general public remain largely unaware of transgender issues, but transgendered individuals are often subject to prejudice, stigma, social injustice, and even violence (Drescher, 2002).

Despite the obvious and apparent mental health needs of these patients, the vast majority of clinicians have little or no formal training in gender issues. It is hoped that this volume can begin a process of correcting that oversight. The goal is to provide useful information for clinicians who are treating, but have little experience with transgendered patients. In addition to educating practitioners about various presentations of transgender subjectivities, clinicians need to think about appropriate referrals for these patients. For those clinicians who wish to learn more about treating transgendered patients, we strongly advise getting supervision from the appropriate experts. [1]

It is also hoped that this volume will be of interest to the general public and to readers, regardless of their own gender status, interested in the growing field of queer theory.

This volume covers a variety of aspects of the transgender experience, including male-to-female and female-to-male presentations, as well as gender-blending. We are also fortunate to have transgendered authors–most of them professionals themselves–contributing to this collection as well. In choosing to present transgendered subjectivities in this volume, we have taken the position that it is useful to clinicians to sympathetically enter the dilemma of those who feel that their biological gender does not match their psychological gender.

We begin with Griffin Hansbury, MA, MSW's "Sexual TNT: A Transman Tells the Truth About Testosterone," an autobiographical essay about the author's first week on testosterone, whose effects on the female body and mind are powerful, stimulating, and sometimes unnerving. This is followed by "The Psychoanalytic Treatment of Gender Dysphoria: A Personal Reflection," a contribution by a transsexual psychiatrist who wishes to remain anonymous. In this personal and moving account, she tells of several unsuccessful psychotherapeutic attempts to resolve her gender dysphoria prior to her sex-reassignment surgery.

The subject then shifts from the personal to the theoretical with Dallas Denny, MA's "Changing Models of Transsexualism." Denny's previous contribution to the journal (2002) is an invaluable resource for those wishing to research the transgender literature. In this issue, she describes changing models of transsexualism, from those which viewed it as a form of mental illness to a new model which explains transsexualism as a natural form of human variability. Her paper discusses both models, and touches on the social and treatment implications of the rise of the newer approach. In another non-pathologizing vein, we also present Aaron Devor, PhD's "Witnessing and Mirroring: A Fourteen Stage Model of Transsexual Identity Formation." Dr. Devor's is an optimistic approach that advocates for acceptance, integration and pride in one's post-transition identity.

From another perspective, Anne Lawrence, MD, PhD, presents "Autogynephilia: A Paraphilic Model of Gender Identity Disorder." Drawing upon the work of Ray Blanchard (1989), Dr. Lawrence explains the little-known (to clinicians) concept of autogynephilia–defined as a male's propensity to be sexually aroused by the thought or image of himself as female. She argues that the idea of autogynephilia–which is conceptualized as both a paraphilia and a sexual orientation–provides an alternative to the traditional model of transsexualism that emphasizes gender identity. The concept is controversial to many in the transsexual community, particularly as seen in many of the internet responses to a recent book addressing autogynephilia by J. Michael Bailey (2000). Dr. Lawrence's thoughtful approach to the subject will hopefully cast more light than heat in what is likely to be an ongoing debate.

The bridge from theoretical issues to clinical ones is made by Vernon A. Rosario, MD, PhD, in " 'Qué joto bonita!': Transgender Negotiations of Sex and Ethnicity." A valued member of our editorial board, Dr. Rosario reviews the nosological history of gender atypicality, from nineteenth century "sexual inversion" to transvestitism and transsexualism. He examines how deviations of gender identity, gender role, sexual object, and sexual aim were often collapsed together and how these imbrications continue to persist in both the medical and popular literature on transsexualism. As the role of ethnicity has been especially neglected in the development of gender and sexual identity, he provides case material gathered from a dynamic psychotherapy with a Latina, transgendered sex worker to examine the articulations of ethnicity, gender, and sexuality in both the transgendered subject and her heterosexually-identified male partners.

Continuing in a clinical vein is David Seil, MD's "The Diagnosis and Treatment of Transgendered Patients." He describes the diagnosis and treatment of 271 transgendered patients to reveal four distinct groups not specified in the current *DSM-IV-TR*. Dr. Seil feels these characteristics are important because they determine the internal and external difficulties the patients present to the clinician.

Next is Leah Schaefer, EdD and Connie Wheeler, PhD's "Guilt in Cross Gender Identity Conditions: Presentation and Treatment." While developing psychometric measurements of guilt in gender identity conditions in adults, the authors noted recurring themes in virtually all clients in their clinical practice over the past 25 years. The authors gathered data from both clinical experience and from research studies specifically designed to identify areas in which patients reported feelings of guilt. Data on 787 patients found thirteen themes of guilt in their subjects. The authors believe that understanding the primary sources of the special kind of guilt connected with gender dysphoria is crucial to understanding the gender dysphoric person.

"Disclosure, Risks and Protective Factors for Children Whose Parents Are Undergoing a Gender Transition," by Tonya White, MD, and Randi Ettner, PhD, is a study which attempts to delineate the effects of a parent's undergoing a transition to the other sex on children at different stages of development. They found that children in the preschool years were rated as adapting best to the transition, both initially and over time, and that adolescents had the most difficult time adapting to a parental transition. They also found that the level of family conflict worsened a child's adaptation across all developmental levels. The authors then go on to delineate both risk and protective factors for children during such a situation.

Charles Ihlenfeld, MD's "Harry Benjamin and Psychiatrists" offers historical perspective on the pioneering physician who founded the transgender field and coined the term "transsexual." Benjamin drew criticism from some in the psychiatric community when he began treating transgendered people with cross-gender hormones and offered encouragement in their efforts in transitioning. By and large, psychiatrists of this time considered gender dysphoria as a manifestation of significant psychopathology and considered the treatment Benjamin was then prescribing as psychiatrically contraindicated. Rather than discouraging Benjamin, this response simply reinforced his feeling that psychiatry as a discipline lacked "common sense." Dr. Ihlenfeld worked for six years with Harry Benjamin, and in his fascinating account, he sketches the development of his own ideas on transgender phenomena.

The volume closes with Irene Willis' "Pronouns," a poem in which the parent of a transgendered person sidesteps all clinical concerns to speak in purely human terms.

The collecting of this diverse content, while striving to maintain editorial consistency, has been challenging. Furthermore, it has taken courage on the part of some of our contributors to disclose personal information about painful and intensely affect-laden private experiences. The editors thank all the contributors for their patience and hard work in bringing this project to fruition. Special thanks are due to Lawrence Soucy, without whose editorial assistance this project would not have been completed. It is our hope that this volume will prove useful in fostering a deeper understanding of gender and–on a deeper level–of human nature.

Ubaldo Leli, MD
Jack Drescher, MD

NOTE

1. Most of the few specialists in the field are affiliated with the Harry Benjamin International Gender Dysphoria Association (HBIGDA). For further information about HBIGDA, contact Bean Robinson, PhD, Executive Director, South Second Street, Suite 180, Minneapolis, MN 55454 USA, Tel: 1-612-625-1500, Fax: 1-612-626-8311, E-mail: *hbigda@famprac.umn.edu*

REFERENCES

Bailey, J. M. (2003), *The Man Who Would Be Queen: The Science of Gender-Bending and Transsexualism.* Washington, DC: Joseph Henry Press.

Blanchard, R. (1989), The concept of autogynephilia and the typology of male gender dysphoria. *J. Nerv. Ment. Dis.*, 177:616-623.

Denny, D. (2002), A selective bibliography of transsexualism. *J. Gay & Lesbian Psychother.*, 6(2):35-66.

Devor, H. (2002), Who are "we"? Where sexual orientation meets gender identity. *J. Gay & Lesbian Psychother.*, 6(2):5-21.

Drescher, J. (2002), An interview with GenderPAC's Riki Wilchens. *J. Gay & Lesbian Psychother.*, 6(2):67-85.

Sexual TNT:
A Transman Tells the Truth
About Testosterone

Griffin Hansbury, MA, MSW

SUMMARY. The following autobiographical essay covers the events and emotions of the author's first week on testosterone in July of 1995, when, at the age of 24, he began his journey from female to male. In the years since, the number of female-to-male transsexuals (FTMs, transmen, etc.) has grown considerably and many of them seek counseling and support from social service agencies and private practitioners, especially in the early days of their transitions. Transition is, in many ways, a second adolescence, both a joyful and stress-filled time. The effects of testosterone on the female body and mind are powerful, stimulating, and sometimes unnerving. This essay provides a behind-the-scenes glimpse into one transman's experience. *[Article copies available for a fee from The Haworth Document Delivery Service: 1-800-HAWORTH. E-mail address: <docdelivery@haworthpress.com> Website: <http://www.HaworthPress.com> © 2004 by The Haworth Press, Inc. All rights reserved.]*

Griffin Hansbury, a former counselor at the Gender Identity Project in New York City, is a graduate of the Hunter College School of Social Work and a Fellow of the New York University School of Medicine's Psychoanalytic Institute. His memoir, *Transman: My Life on Testosterone*, is forthcoming.

Address correspondence to: Griffin Hansbury, MA, MSW, 86 East 7 Street, #5, New York, NY 10003 (E-mail: ghansbury@earthlink.net).

[Haworth co-indexing entry note]: "Sexual TNT: A Transman Tells the Truth About Testosterone." Hansbury, Griffin. Co-published simultaneously in *Journal of Gay & Lesbian Psychotherapy* (The Haworth Medical Press, an imprint of The Haworth Press, Inc.) Vol. 8, No. 1/2, 2004, pp. 7-18; and: *Transgender Subjectivities: A Clinician's Guide* (ed: Ubaldo Leli, and Jack Drescher) The Haworth Medical Press, an imprint of The Haworth Press, Inc., 2004, pp. 7-18. Single or multiple copies of this article are available for a fee from The Haworth Document Delivery Service [1-800-HAWORTH, 9:00 a.m. - 5:00 p.m. (EST). E-mail address: docdelivery@haworthpress.com].

http://www.haworthpress.com/web/JGLP
© 2004 by The Haworth Press, Inc. All rights reserved.
Digital Object Identifer: 10.1300/J236v08n01_02

KEYWORDS. Female-to-male, FTM, male gaze, sex change, sex drive, sexual reassignment, testosterone, transman, transsexual

My mother claims to know the very night I was conceived. When I ask her how she could be so sure, she gets a devilish look and replies, "That night was especially wild," remembering a time when she and my father were still passionate about each other–a time before I existed, a time I can't even imagine. It must have been a hot and humid night; steamy summertime in Massachusetts. My parents went out to see *Man of La Mancha* at the South Shore Music Circus. Under the yellow- and white-striped tent, all aglow in the purple dusk, Don Quixote sang, "To Dream the Impossible Dream." Maybe the egg I used to be was listening at that moment, as it made its way down through the soft tunnels of my mother's body–where the music echoed through its tiny chamber, suggesting the impossible–because my parents went to bed that night, and in their moment of passion, made me.

Impossible or not, I came into the world in pretty much the usual way. I had ten fingers, ten toes, and everything looked normal. I was a healthy female. If there was any indication that I would one day grow up to become a man, it was not evident at my birth. There were no undescended testicles lurking in the translucent depths of my lower half, no enlarged clitoris that would inspire the doctor's silver-quick trimming. If my testosterone levels were too high, or my prolactin levels were too low; if my corpus callosum–the bridge that spans the two hemispheres of the brain–was narrower, like a male's, nobody could see it. If I had a soul shivering in that small, slippery-new body, and it was the soul of a boy, it was invisible then.

I don't have the answer that will cut the Gordian knot of how a person like me comes to be, via culture or biology. I like to believe that we enter this world as sentient souls, dressed in the unshakeable habits of our bodies. Once here, we are influenced by the shapes of those bodies, both inside and out. Inside, our own unique alchemy of hormones, chromosomes, and brain cells conspire to shape our behaviors and tastes. While on the outside, our bodies move through a world of Objects and Others, of circumstances, and blind luck–additional forces that push and pull us along multiple paths.

The etiology of transsexuality is a question I have stopped asking, for myself and for my practice. We're here–now what? That is the question. For me, after 24 years of living uncomfortably in my female body, the answer was to transition. And so I took the usual first steps; I began the psychotherapy required by the Harry Benjamin Standards of Care and then started taking testosterone.

Testosterone is a powerful chemical. Its production turned on by the Y chromosome in utero, it changes otherwise female fetuses into males. Its molecular structure is almost identical to that of estrogen, but for the one extra carbon atom in testosterone. Take away that carbon atom, and you've got estrogen. Men and women both produce testosterone, but men make about ten times as much as women. The normal testosterone range for a human male is 300 to 1,000 nanograms per deciliter of blood; for a female, it is 40 to 60 nanograms per deciliter. Before I began the injections my T level was 49 ng/dl, right smack in the middle of the female average; nothing unusual about that.

Today, immediately following an injection, my testosterone level can soar to a whopping 2,208 ng/dl before falling off to a much more manageable 407 ng/dl, just before the next injection. At my maximum level, I have more than twice as much testosterone as the high-normal male–that's like having the testosterone of two football players racing through my bloodstream.

In my medicine cabinet is a little white box that contains a vial of testosterone cypionate. The box is marked with a day-glo orange sticker that shows a cartoon stick of dynamite and says: "Controlled substance. Dangerous unless used as directed. Federal law prohibits the transfer of this drug to any person other than the patient for whom it was prescribed." The fuse on the cartoon stick of dynamite is lit. If I were to sell this vial, or give it away, I would be committing a felony. Testosterone, they want us to know, is hot stuff. In fact, when the hormone was first synthesized by scientists in 1935, it was hailed as "medical dynamite" and "sexual TNT" (Blum, 1997, p. 159).

Inside the little white box is a pamphlet, written by the folks at Pharmacia & Upjohn in Kalamazoo, Michigan. In it, they describe the drug, its pharmacology, indications, contraindications, warnings, precautions, adverse reactions, etc. "Endogenous androgens," it says, "are responsible for normal growth and development of the male sex organs and for maintenance of secondary sex characteristics." This testosterone solution is indicated for replacement therapy in males with hypogonadism. It is contraindicated for females, who are warned about the serious potential for hirsutism, baldness, vocal cord thickening, clitoral growth, and the litany goes on. The pamphlet does not mention anything about testosterone's power to re-wire the female brain, to actually change the way you think, and the way you see the world.

Testosterone affects a vast array of behaviors and ways of thinking. Football players, blue-collar workers, firefighters, and actors tend to be higher in testosterone than most men and women. Violent criminals have more T than non-violent criminals. People with higher testosterone have more sex partners and they smile less than people with lower testosterone. The hormone is related to navigation, spatial abilities, and travel. "After testosterone injections," writes James M. Dabbs, a cognitive psychologist and expert on testosterone and behavior, "birds travel farther, and mice are less afraid to enter new and strange places." It affects mental rotation ability, the facility to visualize objects from various angles. "People who do well on mental rotation tests should have an advantage when it comes to throwing spears, chipping stone axes, using maps, and repairing carburetors." Dabbs continues, "Females who receive testosterone injections in preparation for sex-change operations show large increases in mental rotation ability" (2000, pp. 52-53).

As I rode the subway home from the doctor's office after that first injection, I worried if, under the influence of testosterone, my brain would become that of a caveman. The human brain has not evolved in 125,000 years. It is the same brain that walked out of Africa several millennia ago, before the invention of agriculture, Eli Whitney's cotton gin, the cellular phone. You can dress a man in a suit and tie, give him a college diploma, a Bible, and an understanding of the theory of relativity, and his brain will still work the way it did back on the Paleolithic veldt, when his male ancestors chipped stone axes and hunted with spears.

I feared that I might turn into a hairy, heavy-browed early *Homo sapiens* who, after the cartoon image, would spend his time clubbing women over the head and dragging them back to his Pleistocene cave, to rut and grunt and scratch amongst the litter of woolly mammoth bones. Would I be transformed into a brutish Stanley Kowalski, who (in the words of Blanche Dubois) "acts like an animal, has an animal's habits! Eats like one, moves like one, talks like one" (Williams, 1971, p. 323)? As much as I might like to look like Marlon Brando circa 1951, I did not want to turn into his rapacious alter ego. Would I become violent? Short-tempered? Short-lived? ("Male birds injected with testosterone sing more, patrol larger areas, have more fights, and are less likely to live out the year," writes Dabbs [p. 36].) And, perhaps worst of all, would I lose my grip on words–the verbal part of my brain shriveling in the hot bath of testosterone? Would I stop writing? Would my writing change? Would I no longer be a writer? What would I become?

That first night of my physical transition, as I lay sleeping with a truckload of testosterone buzzing inside of me, I had a dream that I was being chased by a little girl. She looked like me; or, rather, like the way I looked when I was small. Like the Sunbeam Bread girl, with strawberry-blonde curls and pink cheeks. In the dream, I was hiding in my mother's bedroom, terrified. The Sunbeam girl was trying to break down the door and I was holding it back against her. I was shouting for someone to help, to call Bellevue to come get her and lock her up. *She* was the crazy one; not me. At last, an ambulance came and two men dressed in white took her away. She was surprisingly relaxed when she went, actually limp. She did not struggle as the men strapped her to a gurney, put a blue ice-pack over her, and pushed her into the ambulance, which I thought look like an ice-cream truck, white and cold. I stood watching while the ambulance drove away, with that little girl inside, and there was a sadness to the dream, mixed with a great sense of relief.

I woke the next morning with the dream lingering about me, like a vapor of perfume left by someone who has just stepped out of the room, and I felt that mixture of sadness and relief that the dream had stirred up. The meaning of the dream seemed obvious. But was she really gone, that girlish shadow that chased after me? Had I changed overnight? Had the shot of testosterone that was right then riding the tangled circuitry of my bloodstream turned me, like Kafka's Samsa, into a new creature–perhaps even a monster–just over the course of the past eight hours? I lay in bed and put my hand to my face, feeling my cheeks for the rough stubble of beard. There was none; my cheeks were as smooth and bare as they had been the day before; as they had always been. I got out of bed and went to the bathroom. I hesitated before looking into the mirror. Would I recognize myself? What if there was suddenly a man in there? But I was exactly the same. I inspected my face for the slightest change–a single new hair, a roughness to the skin–but there was none. And again I felt a mixture of sadness and relief. Sadness, because I wanted the changes to hurry up; and relief, because the idea of rushing headlong into manhood was a dream almost too frightening to come true.

I got dressed for the first day at my new job. I had, only two months before, completed a master's degree in Creative Writing and now I was embarking on a career in publishing. I had an idealized, 1950s vision of what publishing would be like, with men in tweedy suits and sexy, smart women in black skirts and horn-rimmed glasses. Everyone would drink martinis at lunch and talk about nothing but capital-L Literature. Working as an editorial assistant in the College Textbook Division of a major publisher, however, would prove to be very different.

On that first day, I dressed in a new pair of khakis and a blue oxford shirt. The office was casual; thankfully, I would not have to negotiate the labyrinth of professional dress, with its strictly gendered skirts and pantyhose vs. suits and ties. Khakis and an oxford shirt were sufficiently gender neutral, so that when I walked in to the office that morning, I am sure, everyone saw me as a lesbian. My hair was short, I walked like a man, sat like a man. I was, for all observers, butch. No one could see the new chemical I had racing through my body. I was filled with far more testosterone than any man in that office, and nobody knew it.

The night after my first day at work, I sat at home, basking in the success of my first day on testosterone. That's when the hot flashes hit me. In an instant, I was dripping in sweat. My throat felt like it was closing up. I couldn't breathe. My heart was pounding against my rib-cage. The testosterone, I was sure, was killing me. I lay down on my couch, convinced I was having a heart attack. No, I was having a aneurysm. The hormone was going straight to my brain and driving me crazy. I remembered a show I'd seen as a kid, an After School Special about a girl who took too much Angel Dust. She went crazy and jumped out the window. "I am not going crazy, I am not going crazy, I am not going crazy," I repeated out loud to myself and tried to relax with some deep breathing exercises. My heart kept bumping along. I could feel it in my throat, ga-thump, ga-thump, ga-thump. I regressed to the Catholicism of my childhood and prayed to the Virgin Mary, the blessed Mother. I thought about stopping my transition.

No one really knows what long-term effects exogenous testosterone has on the female body. There just aren't enough aged female-to-male transsexuals to do any complete studies. What we do understand, at this time, is that transmen run the same risks as average, non-transsexual males. That means that the testosterone will probably shorten my natural life-span. Like any man, I am not expected to outlive my female contemporaries. By undertaking this transition, I have potentially clipped a decade off the end of my life. With my blood pressure raised, my risk of heart disease is increased. My risk of stroke is increased. I have to exercise regularly, watch my diet, my cholesterol, and triglycerides, not smoke or drink too much, and take special care of my liver.

I lay on my couch that night, trembling and sweating, and thinking about all these risks. I imagined the testosterone zipping through my body, setting my blood on fire, tearing through my organs. I wanted to make it stop. I didn't want to do it anymore. I didn't want to spend the rest of my life having to shoot myself up every few weeks, just to lie on my couch sweating and trembling and praying to the Virgin Mary. I thought I was going to die and that would have been just fine. Live as a man, or die. I had no other options.

After about two hours, the palpitations subsided and I relaxed and went to bed. That was the only time the testosterone affected me that way. I don't know why I had such an extreme reaction; no other transman I've spoken to experienced anything similar. I called my endocrinologist the next day, and he told me it was "just anxiety," perhaps coupled with the testosterone's sudden spiking of my blood pressure. Under my skin, a storm was raging. Now I knew I was changing. Deep down in the dark fibers of my body, a revolution was taking place. And, although it was still invisible, it had just shown that it would not be quiet.

I got that first injection on July 10, 1995. Only six days later, I wrote in my diary, "My voice is changing, deepening. Already I can feel it in the back of my throat. It cracks and I cannot sing." My vocal chords were thickening. I had to keep clearing my throat. People asked me, "Are you getting a cold?" I had a frog in my throat. I couldn't believe it was happening so quickly. The onset of the physical changes is different for everyone; for me, it took an amazing six days.

With the physical changes came the emotional and psychological. All of a sudden, everything was sexual. It was as if the whole world had turned into Vegas and Times Square rolled into one, as if everything I encountered–from books to food to human beings—held up a neon sign, a red triple-X to quicken my blood and lure me closer. I got excited just standing up against the Xerox machine at work, making endless copies of manuscripts on that warm, shuddering inanimate object. The sight of a red convertible racing down Fifth Avenue could send a jolt through my pants. But it was on the subway where I felt most vulnerable to my newly super-charged libido. In the jostling and shoving, the rhythmic rush of the train hurtling suggestively through its dark tunnel; in the midst of all the women crammed inside, lightly sweating beneath the fragrance of their shampooed hair in the mornings, I was reduced to a single-minded animal, panting with desire, unable to think of anything but sex.

The way I thought about sex was different than the way I used to. Before testosterone, if I rode the subway and saw an attractive woman, I would think first, "She's attractive. I like her hair, her skirt, her eyes." I thought first in words. My mind was full of language, and from that language would come a narrative. I told myself a story in which I spoke to the girl, asked her name, and how was that book she was reading? After that, the story progressed to our first date, during which there might be dancing, some flirting, conversation, and then kissing, and then—only after the story had spun itself out in detail (what she was wearing, what I was wearing, what music was playing)—we would have sex. And that part, too steamy even for an R-rating, often happened offscreen. The camera in my mind would cut from the kiss straight away to the post-coital cigarette, as it were, when the real live girl got off at 34th Street or Bleecker, and my subway ride continued chastely on.

After testosterone, it was very different. I'd see a woman on the train—she needn't even be attractive to me—if she had a shapely calf, or a knee bared above knee-high socks; if she wore a low-cut shirt that showed the tops of her breasts, or a cropped top that bared her tanned midriff, it was enough. The rest of her could be unappealing. It didn't matter now because I had acquired the ability to separate women into pieces, to dismember them so that all I saw was an arm, a leg, an ankle—the sight of which stuffed my brain instantly with pornographic images. My safe and familiar narrative was usurped by flashes of flesh colors, brute photographs, reels of dirty movies at which I stared mindlessly enrapt, without thought, in a sort of pre-verbal daze.

The images came without invitation, and I could not stop them. My desire became enormous— and it brought with it a physical response as well. When I looked at a woman, I got an erection. The female body has its own share of erectile tissue, and mine was responding to the flood of testosterone—the hormone responsible, in males and females, for engorging the genitals with blood during sexual arousal; more testosterone means more blood-flow, and that equals bigger, harder penises and clitorises. In addition, the clitoris grows considerably longer and fatter under the influence of extra androgens, until it resembles a very small penis. I began to understand the drive in men, pulled by that divining rod between their legs, to press forward. While the images flickered and burned inside my brain, there was nothing cognitive about it. It was utterly, devastatingly physical. At the sight of a woman's legs, breasts, arms, whatever, the desire was instantaneous and unstoppable. I wanted to grab her and push my way into her.

As the days passed after my first injection, my sex drive kept climbing, until I could think of nothing else. My brain was a 24-hour pornographic cinema, in which images of naked women bombarded my thoughts without pause. It was unbearably distracting. How do teenage boys ever survive the drudgery of algebra, Shakespeare, the Industrial Revolution, with this endless reel of pornography flooding their brains? I was 24 years old, and I could hardly do my work.

At the office, I sat at my desk reading a manuscript for a Freshman Composition literature anthology. The open pages of the manuscript became the open legs of a girl, a pair of thighs, pale and smooth. Blotting out the text of a Maya Angelou poem, there arose lurid images of split-open melons, honeydews, the juice glistening in their middles. I couldn't stop thinking of women's bodies as pieces of fruit. I couldn't walk past a fruit stand without seeing women's body parts in its display. My sexual urgings became a cliché of what I believed was "typical male" desire. I felt so tacky and unoriginal. Still, those honeydews, with their pneumatic roundness, their shining wetness, their sticky insides. When you are a man, the whole world conspires to seduce you, grabbing you by the pant-leg and pulling you down a few rungs on the ladder of cultural evolution.

As an undergraduate at Bryn Mawr College, I was a sex-positive, post-feminist, butch dyke. I balked at claims that men are more visually aroused by pornographic images, while women get turned on from reading Harlequin romance novels, "bodice-rippers," Anais Nin's florid erotica. Gender was nothing more than a cultural construction, after all. I was a woman (or so I considered myself at the time), and I enjoyed pornography. In my dorm room I kept a small stash of nudie magazines. I believed then that the pictures gave me a real charge, but it was nothing compared to my reaction post-testosterone.

Before testosterone, I could not understand why men were held in thrall by the sight of a woman, lovely or otherwise endowed with some magnetic quality. I'd watch men on the street and in the subways, watching women with a look of total submission, slack-jawed and starving as if they'd just arrived from some famine-ravaged country and the woman was a four-course meal. It was a look that disgusted me–until I began to wear that same mask of hunger, the infamous "male gaze."

At Bryn Mawr, I was introduced to the concept of the male gaze through the work of feminist film theorist Laura Mulvey. In *Visual and Other Pleasures* she writes, "In a world ordered by sexual imbalance, pleasure in looking has been split between active/male and passive/female. The determining male gaze projects its phantasy onto the female figure, which is styled accordingly. In their traditional exhibitionist role women are simultaneously looked at and displayed, with their appearance coded for strong visual and erotic impact so that they can be said to connote *to-be-looked-at-ness*" (1989, p. 19).

Mulvey uses psychoanalysis and Freud's "scopophilia"–the pleasure of looking, of turning people into objects for sexual arousal–to reveal the inner workings of the "phallocentric cinema." In the decades that have passed since Mulvey's article, feminists have searched for an empowered female gaze, one that is neither narcissistic nor passive–one that converts the male figure into an object to be visually enjoyed. And today, more than ever, the male body is on display. You see his perfected Apollonian physique on billboards, magazine covers, in Coca-Cola commercials. The male body has successfully been turned into erotic spectacle–but not by the female gaze. If anybody turned men into pin-ups, it was other men.

Perhaps there can be no scopophilic female gaze. Not that women don't enjoy looking, but it takes a certain kind of cultural power to convert people into objects, a power that women may never possess. And what's so terrible about being an object anyway? Objects have a tremendous power all their own. Maybe we're going about this all wrong. Perhaps "male" and "female" are inaccurate designations when this Gaze that endows women, and men, with "to-be-looked-at-ness" is fueled by testosterone, a hormone both men and women possess in varying quantities. The "male gaze" may have evolved into an instrument of culture, but its source is purely biological. Better to call it the Testosterone Gaze.

There does not appear to be a cohesive theory as to why men are so much more visually turned on than women, but there are bits and pieces that, once put together, provide a satisfactory explanation–and it all has to do with testosterone.

Testosterone levels, researchers have found, are flexible; they rise and fall in response to different situations. In competition, like a fist-fight or a football game, T rises in the winner and falls in the loser. This holds true even for spectators. At the end of Superbowl Sunday, fans of the winning team receive a spike in their T levels, while those rooting for the losers will take a downturn.[1] These results have been observed in men–and in monkeys, in which T levels remain high in the winner for about 24 hours after a fight, and stay lower in the loser for even longer. However, if the loser catches sight of a "sexually receptive female" (we're talking monkeys here), his testosterone levels get a boost. This sounds not unlike the effect a man might feel while watching strippers in a topless bar; women who are paid to appear "sexually receptive." In fact, reports author Deborah Blum in her book *Sex on the Brain*, "Watching other monkeys have sex–at some level, comparable to strip bars or porno flicks, I suppose–boosts male monkeys' T-levels up some 400 percent" (p. 168). No wonder men like to look.

In addition, evolutionary biology propels (most) males to inseminate as many females as possible, as quickly as possible. This "race to reproduce" requires quick reflexes.

"By theory," writes Blum, "we should see a rapid response to the very sight of a sexually attractive partner. Every study shows that this describes males. There's some evidence, for instance, that testosterone is wired for visual response. T-levels rise in monogamous male birds as they watch a female. Female birds, however, are rarely jazzed by mere sight of the opposite sex. In humans, the male system sometimes seems so jittery with sexual readiness that just about anything–high-heeled shoes, a smile, a friendly conversation–will produce a sexual response" (pp. 227-228).

To that list, I would add: Xerox machines, red convertibles, subway cars.

One dazzling sunny afternoon, in that first week on testosterone, I was walking up Fifth Avenue on my lunch hour when an ass caught my eye–not a woman with an ass, mind you; in my dismembering testosterone gaze it was just an ass–dressed in a tight satiny skirt, decorated with a blossoming rose embroidered on each cheek. As it floated along before me, I became hypnotized by the see-saw rhythm of the roses going up and down and was overcome by the need to see what kind of breasts belonged to such a powerful ass. I quickened my pace and moved in front, when my cultural consciousness kicked in. "Don't turn around," it said. And then another, devilish, voice sneered, "Turn around. Go on. Check 'em out." In this way, I argued with myself for a block or two. But the devil on my shoulder triumphed. I turned around. And the breasts looked good under their pink angora sweater, full and round and pointing straight uptown. But after the thrill of looking wore off, I was overcome by a tremendous, feminist guilt and berated myself for ogling that woman on the street, for acting like such a "typical" male. In those first days, I didn't like the man I was becoming.

The lunch hour ended and I walked back to the office, where I opened the manuscript on my desk, that anthology of U.S. Literature. It was my job to revise the table of contents, but I wasn't in the mood. I felt like reading something–something that would tell me about this new life, and give me some guidance, the way books and stories had always done. I turned to Irwin Shaw's short story "The Girls in Their Summer Dresses," and read it through to the end, fascinated by these words especially:

> When I think of New York City, I think of all the girls . . . all on parade in the city. I don't know whether it's something special with me or whether every man in the city walks around with the same feeling inside him, but I feel as though I am at a picnic in this city . . . when the warm

weather comes, the girls in their summer dresses . . . I can't help but look at them. I can't help but want them. (1984, p. 67)

I couldn't help it either. In those first months of transition, with a few more injections under my belt, my second puberty galloped along and I lived within the body of a teenage boy, balancing on the cusp between wolf and man. Like the werewolf (that symbol of pubertal anxiety), I began to sprout hair all over my body and the smoothness of my face vanished beneath the stubble of a beard. My cracking voice settled into a smooth and resonant baritone. My muscles thickened and my bones grew denser. And eventually, after several months, my raging libido leveled off and mellowed out, enabling me to think again of subjects other than sex.

My journey across the sexes (if there can even be such a thing) turned me–kicking and screaming, at first–towards biological determinism, even though that philosophy seems to stand in direct opposition to transsexuality. If biology were truly destiny, then how could I possibly transcend it as I have? Still, I know, in a visceral way that perhaps only a transsexual man or woman can know, that males and females are different animals, despite their many similarities, and that culture is only part of the reason why–perhaps more a byproduct of biology than an originating force. We can chicken-and-egg the issue all we want, but biology was here first. When we were but single-celled creatures, there was no talk of romance, or pornography, or oppression. There was no talk at all.

Testosterone turned my world on its head. It changed the way I look and the way I am looked at by others. It changed how I think and how I express my thoughts. And it changed the way I see the world. In the beginning, these changes were new and sometimes frightening. It took a long time to adjust. Nearly a decade later, I still haven't learned all the new rules, the social codes of gender that come along when you take on a new biology. Many of those rules I find myself fighting against. Before testosterone, I didn't fit the prescribed role of woman, and today I don't quite fit the role of man, either. If testosterone changed me into a biological determinist, then living every day as a man–with a female history–has turned me into a social constructivist. I suppose, like my own complex gender identity, I inhabit both spheres simultaneously. And, more often than not, I contradict myself. As Walt Whitman said, "I am large, I contain multitudes."

NOTE

1. This may explain the seeming contradiction of triumphant basketball fans rioting in the streets, and the higher rates of domestic violence in the homes of winning football fans: Hopped up on high-T, they explode with aggression. Losers don't have the energy to set fire to cities or beat their wives.

REFERENCES

Blum, D. (1997), *Sex on the Brain: The Biological Differences Between Men and Women*. New York, NY: Penguin Books.

Dabbs, J. (2000), *Heroes, Rogues, and Lovers: Testosterone and Behavior*. New York, NY: McGraw-Hill Publishers.

Mulvey, L. (1989), *Visual and Other Pleasures*. London: Macmillan Press Ltd.

Shaw, I. (1984), *Short Stories: Five Decades*. New York, NY: Delacorte Press.

Williams, T. (1971), *The Theatre of Tennessee Williams, Vol. 1*. New York, NY: New Directions.

The Psychoanalytic Treatment
of Gender Dysphoria:
A Personal Reflection

Anonymous

SUMMARY. The author, a male to female transsexual psychiatrist, provides a personal account of several unsuccessful psychotherapeutic attempts to resolve her gender dysphoria prior to sex-reassignment surgery. *[Article copies available for a fee from The Haworth Document Delivery Service: 1-800-HAWORTH. E-mail address: <docdelivery@haworthpress.com> Website: <http://www.HaworthPress.com> © 2004 by The Haworth Press, Inc. All rights reserved.]*

KEYWORDS. Gender dysphoria, gender identity disorder, psychoanalysis, psychotherapy, transsexual psychiatrist, transsexualism

It is quite strange to reflect on the reality that I was born in 1950 and somehow was unaware of the phenomenon of transsexualism until 1969 or 1970 when I read an article in *Look* magazine describing the lives of individuals who had had sexual reassignment surgery (Christine Jorgensen had her surgery in 1952). Perhaps, I could blame it on growing up in a town in West Texas; but then, I believe that I would be avoiding the reality of denial. Of

---

The author wishes to remain anonymous.

[Haworth co-indexing entry note]: "The Psychoanalytic Treatment of Gender Dysphoria: A Personal Reflection." Anonymous. Co-published simultaneously in *Journal of Gay & Lesbian Psychotherapy* (The Haworth Medical Press, an imprint of The Haworth Press, Inc.) Vol. 8, No. 1/2, 2004, pp. 19-24; and: *Transgender Subjectivities: A Clinician's Guide* (ed: Ubaldo Leli, and Jack Drescher) The Haworth Medical Press, an imprint of The Haworth Press, Inc., 2004, pp. 19-24. Single or multiple copies of this article are available for a fee from The Haworth Document Delivery Service [1-800-HAWORTH, 9:00 a.m. - 5:00 p.m. (EST). E-mail address: docdelivery@haworthpress.com].

course, it is not entirely true to say that I was unaware of the "phenomenon of transsexualism," but all I knew was that I was different and that I was "wrong." I do wish that the anamnesis of the psychoanalytic process would enable me to say with some certainty when I first knew that I was different; unfortunately, it does not. But then, I only gradually became aware of my difference as it was revealed in my interactions with others and reflected back to me. This mirroring certainly let me know of my difference; it was this knowledge and a desire to be "undifferent" that led to my struggles and my depression and my ultimate contact with psychiatry.

I believe that I tried very hard to somehow transform myself into the image that was reflected back to me in my encounters with parental and societal expectations. It was discouraging to recognize again and again that my efforts were failures, at least if I were to believe what was said to me by my playmates and others. My first recollection of being overwhelmed by this sense of being different came when my father relocated us for a year from Texas to New England. Now, in addition to the long-standing difference that shadowed me, I was further marked by the drawl that characterizes speech in Texas. It was one more thing that I had to try to hide. Anything that marked me as being different was not a source of pride, but rather one of shame and embarrassment. The time that I thought that I might be able to truly achieve this hiding myself from both others and myself would not come until much later.

It is not my intention, however, to focus upon my experiences growing up and being gender variant (others have done this quite eloquently and I believe that my experiences are so similar to theirs as to only be a variation on the theme) or how these experiences may have figured in my ultimate decision to attend medical school and to become a psychiatrist. Rather, I would like to focus on the experiences that I have had in my contacts with psychiatrists and psychotherapists, since the mirroring process continued in the psychotherapeutic and psychoanalytic situation in spite of the stance of therapeutic neutrality.

My first contacts with psychiatrists occurred in 1968. At this time, the focus was on my dysthymia (or as it was called at the time, my neurotic depression). Although I knew the issue involved being intensely unhappy due to my gender and the guilt that I felt due to my difference, this was not something that I could bring myself to discuss. I grew up in an environment of physicians who were not particularly psychiatrically minded, and any contact with psychiatry was actively discouraged. It is certainly worth mentioning that the psychiatrist in the student health service at the university in which I was enrolled allowed me to continue my contacts with her beyond the usually allotted time for crisis resolution; and she was perceptive enough to bring up the issue of my gender related unhappiness in a sensitive enough manner that it should have opened the discussion. However, I was unable to accept the invitation from her to do so.

Later, I learned that the issue was difficult enough for me to discuss with a therapist that I had to mention it in the first interview or it might not be discussed at all. My first effort to bring up my gender-related unhappiness with a non-physician therapist led to the following response: if I were talking about something beyond my discomfort with gender role behavior, then I needed to be talking with a psychiatrist. My conclusion from this interaction was that if this were the case, then I was far too disturbed and he would be unable to continue the therapy with me. I learned to keep the discussion within the bounds of what was comfortable for him. Like the character Alan Bates portrays in the movie, *The Shout*, uttering the words of the reality in which I was living might bring about the destruction of my world.

My efforts to explain my conundrum to my next psychiatrist were still without success as the effort was made for me to adjust to my situation and perhaps redefine my gender role expectations in a way that would enable me to be happy with my biological sex. This came at a time when I was in medical school, when I was so convinced of my difference that I was reluctant to have a karyotype done since I was fearful that people would then know of my struggle. I was aware, at least on a preconscious level, that the issue of my identity was fundamental enough that it would be reflected in my chromosomes; I was certain that my karyotype would not be XY.

Still driven by a desire to conform and become "undifferent"–since this is what was being mirrored by all around me, including the one therapist and three psychiatrists that I had thus far consulted–I decided that I would enter into psychoanalysis during my third year of medical school. I had learned enough in my academic career thus far that I had come to the conclusion that this would be the avenue of my escape; that the depth of psychoanalysis would provide me the avenue to leave the prison of difference in which I was trapped. I hoped that I would finally be able to join those around me in the full experience of life and not remain isolated as the mariner in Coleridge's poem who believed that he was unable to enter into the celebration of life in the wedding feast.

As a medical student, I was able to borrow money from the state medical association to finance this experience. I entered into treatment with a training analyst with the New Orleans Analytic Institute. His approach was conservative; I was meeting with him three times a week on the couch and attempting free association. I was given little in the way of reflection or feedback or direction. My analyst's understanding of my gender difficulty was right out of Otto Fenichel: I learned from him that my gender difficulty was a conflict between my ability to accept my being male and an effort to disguise my sexual drive.

The experience of that analysis may have provided me with enough support to enable me to complete medical school, but it wasn't helping me to resolve the issue that had brought me to analysis in the first place. As I had to interrupt the treatment due to lack of funds and graduation from medical school, I then revealed to him my frustration with the lack of resolution. My analyst seemed genuinely surprised that his earlier interpretation hadn't resolved the gender issue for me. As it turns out, I had simply given up the discussion with him; and rather than inquiring further about the subject, my analyst had made the erroneous assumption that the issue had been resolved for me.

Following the medical internship component of my residency, I was able to resume my experience in psychoanalysis, although technically it was initially psychoanalytic psychotherapy on a once-a-week basis, face to face. This decision was driven by financial constraints. My new therapist was a training analyst for the Western New England Psychoanalytic Institute. I entered treatment expressing the desire to become "undifferent," and I was told that he had no reservations about working on this issue with me. Fortunately, his approach was not as conservative as the previous analyst. So, with the completion of my residency, he allowed me to continue with him in psychoanalysis. We met four-times-a-week with me lying on the couch, something I could now financially afford.

There was an occasion when I queried him about his lack of confrontation of the gender issue. He told me that he knew "better than to confront a delusion." Being told that my identity conflict was something that he viewed as delusional left me with the same sense of futility and hopelessness that I had experienced with the interpretation from my previous analyst. These people were training analysts. I believed they held the secrets and the keys to my escape. If they were unable to help me, where else could I turn? I'm sure that this is what kept me engaged with the process; either my belief was delusional or perhaps my belief that there could be some escape was the delusion. I had no choice that I could see but to "trust in the process."

Later, as I was going through a particularly dark period of depression, I commented to my analyst that if I were treating someone as depressed as I was then, I would be prescribing a medication. The next appointment he said that he had thought about my comment and suggested that I start taking an amitriptyline/perphenazine combination. I refused this medication due to the antipsychotic component; I did not believe that I was psychotic.

Despite these experiences, I did gain much from the contact with this analyst, and I managed for a time to completely avoid allowing myself to even think in terms of my gender conflict. This came after a rather intense crisis in a relationship, and I believe that my analyst may have thought that I was "cured." It certainly was evident that he was pleased with my resolution so, when I could no longer continue functioning with this avoidance and suppression, I believed that I had not only failed myself but disappointed him as well. There later came a time when he suggested that I terminate the analysis over the next couple of months. It was my belief at this time that this was his way of saying that my situation was hopeless. Uncertain how I could function if he abandoned me at this point, I was quite discouraged. I told him both that the timing was wrong and that I was motivated to continue–so we did. Perhaps if he had had an understanding of my gender confusion beyond what was theorized by Fenichel, Klein, Balint, Kohut, and all the others, he might have helped me to come to the recognition that my efforts to overcome my "difference" through the psychoanalytic process were futile.

Swimming laps in an otherwise empty pool one evening after work, I was overcome with a sense of terror. I had the fantasy that I was swimming in the pool with a shark. The fantasy was so powerful that it was difficult for me to remain in the pool, despite my attempts to remind myself of the reality of my situation. The next day, while attempting to describe the intensity of the experience to my analyst, he made an off-hand comment that made light of my experience. I was able to express my disappointment that he was unable to recognize the intensity of my fear. It was probably at this point that I realized that I wasn't going to be given the means to escape through any door that psychoanalysis was going to open. Reflecting on this experience today, I realize that it was much like the belief that I had in medical school about my chromosomal makeup. The shark with which I was swimming was the gender issue and I was in danger of being consumed by it.

I had another relationship crisis a few months later in which I realized that my partner was unable to either really understand my gender dilemma or to accept it. I was directed by a family member, with whom I had confided the nature of my identity issue, to a gender support group. I had also decided to terminate my analysis; I had come to a point of acceptance with respect to my identity. Perhaps it wasn't quite acceptance at this point, but resignation to the reality that all of my efforts to somehow escape the reality of my difference that was being mirrored to me had been futile. My analyst told me that the time was not right and that I should take a year to think about it. I was not able to figure out why I had been offered the option of terminating over a period of a few months a year earlier, but now I was being told to take a year to think about the decision to terminate. I decided to set a termination date two months away and continued my contact with the support group. This actually represented the first time that I had had any contact with any other individuals who identified themselves as transgendered.

Being a psychiatrist in the transgender community is often difficult because, for the most part, psychiatrists have been labeled as the enemy. Given psychiatry's general lack of understanding of transgendered phenomena and its historical view of those experiences as arising from a set of dynamic–rather than as something more essential–it is easy to see how this might be. On some level, the prolonged experience of attempts at some kind of reparation was useful in terms of coming to accept who I was rather than trying to change.

Perhaps this resolution came in spite of, rather than because of, the psycho-therapeutic and psychoanalytic contact that I had. Certainly, there is much of what I experienced in psychotherapy and psychoanalysis that has been quite beneficial in terms of the resolution of other issues in my life. I know that the patience of my second analyst in my struggles to sort through the many ways that my gender variance had affected me. That new experience of my self and my place in the world around me afforded me a springboard that enabled me to enter into the world of the TG community. Somehow his comment early in the analysis that "just because something seems to be one way doesn't mean that that is the way that it is" guided me through many situations that I found confusing.

I did subsequently contact the psychologist who was the head of the local gender identity clinic. This contact came when I had finally decided that the course of avoidance was no longer viable. These contacts were quite helpful in affording me a venue to discuss some of the issues involved with the progression of my ultimate transition and sexual reassignment surgery. Being able to approach this transition from a standpoint other than one that assumed some fault in my psychic structure made this possible.

I have had some contact with my last analyst since my transition and genital surgery. He had heard about the process I had undergone, as I had expected he would. When I told him of my current sense of resolution and stability, he said that he would then have to regard the analysis as having been successful. It was clear, however, that he regarded the outcome as being otherwise when he went on to say that we all have dynamics that we need to resolve. Clearly, it would have been better, from his perspective, if I had maintained my state of suppression and functioned heterosexually; his second choice would have been for me to be homosexual; the course I had chosen was a distant third. He may have just been unable to grasp the fact that thinking in terms of psycho-dynamics and conflict theory offered little understanding of transsexualism, although those theories can be useful in understanding what is involved in being transsexual. This latter understanding is the gift that he gave to me.

REFERENCES

Fenichel, O. (1945), *The Psychoanalytic Theory of Neurosis*. New York: Norton.
Jorgensen, C. (1967), *Christine Jorgensen: A Personal Autobiography*. New York: Paul S. Ericksson, Inc. Reprinted in 1968 by Bantam Books.

Changing Models of Transsexualism

Dallas Denny, MA

SUMMARY. The second half of the twentieth century saw the development within the psychological and medical communities of a transsexual
model and procedures for identifying, describing, and treating individuals who sought sex reassignment. This model viewed transsexualism as
a form of mental illness characterized by a pervasive and ongoing wish
to be a member of the other sex. The model prescribes a set of medical
and social procedures called sex reassignment, whereby an individual
"changed sex." The 1990s saw the rise of a new model which explained
transsexualism as a natural form of human variability. This model,
which continues to gain prominence, views sex reassignment as but one
of a variety of acceptable life choices for transsexual individuals, and
recognizes the need and right of nontranssexual transgendered people to
make similar choices. This paper discusses both models and touches on
the social and treatment implications of the rise of the transgender
model. *[Article copies available for a fee from The Haworth Document Delivery Service: 1-800-HAWORTH. E-mail address: <docdelivery@haworthpress.com>
Website: <http://www.HaworthPress.com> © 2004 by The Haworth Press, Inc.
All rights reserved.]*

KEYWORDS. Cross dresser, *DSM*, gender dysphoria, gender identity
disorder, gender-variant, HIV, sex reassignment, transgender, transsexual

---

Dallas Denny is the editor of *Transgender Tapestry*, and the Executive Director of
the American Educational Gender Information Service, Inc.
Address correspondence to: Dallas Denny, MA, P.O. Box 33724, Decatur, GA
30033-0724 (E-mail: aegis@gender.org).

[Haworth co-indexing entry note]: "Changing Models of Transsexualism." Denny, Dallas. Co-published
simultaneously in *Journal of Gay & Lesbian Psychotherapy* (The Haworth Medical Press, an imprint of The
Haworth Press, Inc.) Vol. 8, No. 1/2, 2004, pp. 25-40; and: *Transgender Subjectivities: A Clinician's Guide*
(ed: Ubaldo Leli, and Jack Drescher) The Haworth Medical Press, an imprint of The Haworth Press, Inc.,
2004, pp. 25-40. Single or multiple copies of this article are available for a fee from The Haworth Document
Delivery Service [1-800-HAWORTH, 9:00 a.m. - 5:00 p.m. (EST). E-mail address: docdelivery@
haworthpress.com].

http://www.haworthpress.com/web/JGLP
© 2004 by The Haworth Press, Inc. All rights reserved.
Digital Object Identifer: 10.1300/J236v08n01_04

Transsexualism was defined in the mid-20th century as a condition in which an individual wishes to manifest the primary and secondary sex characteristics of the non-natal sex and live as a member of that sex, and modifies his or her body with hormones and surgery to achieve that end (Benjamin, 1966; American Psychiatric Association, 1980). The 1990s, however, brought an increasing awareness among researchers and clinicians that genital sex reassignment surgery (SRS) is not uniformly desired or sought by all persons who dress and behave as members of the other sex on a full-time basis. This new paradigm (Denny, 1995) originating from transgendered people themselves (see especially Prince, 1973, and Boswell, 1991), provided an alternative to the model of transsexualism which had held sway since the 1960s (see Benjamin, 1966; Green and Money, 1969). The initial model held that transsexuals were "trapped in the wrong body," experiencing a psychic pain that could be alleviated only by body transformation. The new model views gender as a continuum rather than a male/female dichotomy (Bornstein, 1994; Rothblatt, 1994) and calls for individualized gender trajectories, which may or may not include hormonal therapy and sex reassignment surgery.

By the mid-1990s, the term transgender[ed] was widely used to describe all persons whose identities, behavior, or dress varied from traditional gender norms–not only transsexuals, transgenderists, crossdressers, and drag queens, but also those who challenged clothing or occupational norms, even gay men and lesbians, who transgress the norms of sexual attraction (cf Bornstein, 1994). Today, the transgender model is reflected not only in the lay and professional literatures, but in the *DSM IV* (American Psychiatric Association, 1994), in which the diagnostic category Transsexualism was replaced with the more general Gender Identity Disorder (GID); and in the proceedings of the Harry Benjamin International Gender Dysphoria Association,[1] which named its electronic periodical, *The International Journal of Transgenderism*.

DEVELOPMENT OF THE TRANSSEXUAL MODEL

In his seminal work *The Transsexual Phenomenon* (1966), Harry Benjamin, who had worked with hundreds of men and women desperate to change their sex, defined a syndrome he called *transsexualism*. Transsexuals were those men and women who were psychologically and socially a poor fit in their assigned sex, and who wished to belong to the other sex. Perhaps the defining characteristic was misery. Transsexuals were desperately unhappy in their skins. Some of these individuals, Benjamin argued, could be given a measure of relief by providing the medical treatment needed to enable them to live as members of the non-natal sex.

Also in 1966, a gender program was established at Johns Hopkins University. Three years later, Green and Money published a text with chapters representing the wide range of disciplines the Hopkins program used to help transsexuals with the physical, psychological, and social aspects of the process the authors called "sex reassignment." Other clinics soon opened in the U.S., following the multidisciplinary Hopkins model.

The transsexual model was primarily a medical one; it held that transsexualism was a form of mental illness. It was variously argued that the desire to change sex was caused by repressed or denied homosexuality (Socarides, 1969), perversion (Wiedeman, 1953), masochism (Wiedeman, 1953), neurosis (Ostow, 1953), psychosis (Baastrup, 1966), character or personality disorder (Spensley and Barter, 1971), brain trauma (Blumer, 1969), or an attempt by the [male] medical establishment to render females obsolete (Raymond, 1979). Theories of causation ranged from individual psychopathology to family pathology to prenatal, perinatal, or postnatal hormone disturbances or chromosomal aberrations (see Hoenig, 1985 for a review).

Yet the transsexual model provided a medical rationale for procedures which alleviated the suffering of transsexuals. The proponents argued, reasonably, that since no other treatment had been shown effective, sex reassignment should be considered–but only in the most serious and persistent cases: ". . . my principal argument was that we doctors should be as conservative as possible in advising sex-reassignment surgery or in performing such an irrevocable operation . . ." (Benjamin, 1969, p. 6).

The treatment was palliative. The individual would not be cured, but merely rendered able to participate more fully in life's rich banquet (see Green, 1969, p. 471).

> Over the years, psychiatrists have tried repeatedly to treat these people without surgery, and the conclusion is inescapable that psychotherapy has not so far solved the problem. The patients have no motivation for psychotherapy and do not want to change back to their biological sex . . . If the mind cannot be changed to fit the body, then perhaps we should consider changing the body to fit the mind. (John E. Hoopes, quoted in Green and Money, 1969, p. 268)

The opponents of sex reassignment argued that the proper way to deal with a diseased mind was to treat the brain; to do otherwise constituted collaboration with the mental illness: "The difficulty of getting the patient into psychiatric treatment should not lead us to compliance with the patient's demands, which are based on his sexual perversion" (Wiedeman, 1953, responding to Hamburger et al.'s [1953] announcement of the sex reassignment of Christine Jorgensen).

ADVANTAGES OF THE TRANSSEXUAL MODEL

The transsexual model provided a theoretical framework for sex reassignment in an earlier era. It protected transsexuals, who now had a medical problem rather than a moral problem, and it gave professionals a logical reason for treating and studying gender-variant persons: they were doing their duty as healers. Under the auspices of the model, thousands of transsexuals who had previously had nowhere to turn found help.

The medically-based transsexual model brought professionals together to form a community. It made previously unavailable sex reassignment technologies available to transsexuals. The model stimulated much research and the publication of dozens of books and hundreds of articles in professional journals. Without it, there would have been no gender clinics, and the thousands of transsexuals who attended the clinics in the 1960s and 1970s would have been forced to choose between going without treatment or seeking out problematic and often dangerous black market hormones and surgeries.

DISADVANTAGES OF THE TRANSSEXUAL MODEL

Most of the professionals writing in the 1960s and 1970s realized sex reassignment was an extreme treatment which paid homage to bipolar gender norms. Pauly (1969) wrote ". . . we must discard the biblical polarity of the male-female, masculine-feminine dichotomy, and reorient our thinking along a scale of subtle nuances of behavior."

Unfortunately, society was not yet ready to acknowledge that gender comes in shades of grey. Both transsexuals and the professionals who treated them had little choice but to function as best they could within the confines of a world that saw gender as black-and-white, male or female. The transsexual model was well suited for the times.

The model provided the theoretical framework necessary to provide medical treatment to transsexuals, but at a price: the treatment it prescribed–sex reassignment–was predicated on the notion that there were but two genders, and was thus relatively inflexible. Sex reassignment converted males into females and females into males; applicants were either accepted for sex reassignment or turned away; there was no middle ground.

Because treatment was predicated on the notion that the individual was changing sex, most gender clinics rejected those who didn't want SRS as "nontranssexual" (cf Newman and Stoller, 1974). Those accepted into the gender programs often had to fulfill elaborate requirements in order to obtain hormonal therapy and SRS (see Lothstein, 1983, pp. 87-91).

The treatment programs aggressively enforced binary male/female gender norms; those deemed appropriate for sex reassignment were expected and often required to behave and dress in ways that reflected the most extreme masculine and feminine presentations (Bolin, 1988; Denny, 1992). Sometimes, emphasis was placed not only on the ability to successfully pass as a member of the other gender, but on youth and sexual attractiveness:

> A clinician during a panel session on transsexualism said he was more convinced of the femaleness of a male-to-female transsexual if she was particularly beautiful and was capable of evoking in him those feelings that beautiful women generally do. Another clinician told us that he uses his own sexual interest as a criterion for deciding whether a transsexual is really the gender she/he claims. (Kessler and McKenna, 1978, p. 113)

> Most who were rejected for surgery looked like men trying unsuccessfully to imitate women. (Stone, 1977)

Under the transsexual model, the clinics attempted to turn out well-adjusted, attractive, heterosexual graduates. Applicants were rejected for a variety of reasons, including age, sexual orientation, marital status, occupational choice, and projected appearance in the new gender role (Denny, 1992). Even in the mid-1990s, gender programs around the world were turning down applicants for sex reassignment for such reasons (Petersen and Dickey, 1995).

Not surprisingly, transsexuals learned to tell stories consistent with the expectations of their caregivers:

> It took a surprisingly long time–several years–for the researchers to realize that the reason the candidates' behavioral profiles matched Benjamin's so well was that the candidates, too, had read Benjamin's book, which was passed from hand to hand within the transsexual community, and they were only too happy to provide the behavior that led to acceptance for surgery. (Stone, 1991)

> The preoperative individual recognizes the importance of fulfilling caretaker expectations in order to receive a favorable recommendation for surgery, and this may be the single most important factor responsible for the prevalent mental-health medical conceptions of transsexualism. *Transsexuals feel that they cannot reveal information at odds with caretaker expectations without suffering adverse consequences.* They freely admitted to lying to their caretakers about sexual orientation and other issues.
>
> Although caretakers are often aware that transsexuals will present information carefully manipulated to ensure surgery. . . they have only to scrutinize several of their most prominent diagnostic markers available in the literature to realize the reason for the deceit. If caretakers would divorce themselves from these widely held beliefs, they would probably receive more honest information. (Bolin, 1988, p. 63)

It was an unfortunate fact that treatment under the model punished transsexuals for telling the truth. It also placed them at risk for abuse from professionals who controlled access to hormones and SRS. Transsexuals have long complained about this. The literature documents the excesses of the gender programs, some of which required their transsexual clients to divorce, change their names, quit their jobs, dress and behave in stereotypically masculine or feminine ways, and agree to participate in follow-up studies by offering the promise of hormonal therapy and SRS. Stone (1977, p. 142) wrote "All transsexual patients receiving hormone therapy at the clinic were asked to submit to a semi-structured interview, including a medical history, and a problem-specific physical examination. *Participation in the study was mandatory if the patients wished to continue to receive hormone therapy at the clinic*" (emphasis added; see also Denny, 1992).

THE TRANSGENDER MODEL

In 1973, Virginia Prince published an essay questioning the inevitability of SRS for those who lived as members of the non-natal sex. She wrote:

> We have sexual identity clinics in which people are examined, selected, screened, and finally have surgery performed on them . . . It seems a very sad thing to me that a great many individuals have to go to the expense, pain, danger, and everything else when they could achieve a gender change without any of it. (Prince, 1973, p. 21)

In 1991, Boswell provided a theoretical framework for Prince's lived experience:

> . . . in the vast majority of instances, we are not so much "gender conflicted" as we are at odds–even at war–with our culture. It is our culture that imposes the polarization of gender according to biology. It is our culture that has brainwashed us, and our families and friends, who might otherwise be able to love us and embrace our diversity as desirable and natural–something to be celebrated. (Boswell, 1991, p. 30)

Under the transgender model proposed by Boswell, transsexualism and other forms of gender variance are viewed not as mental disorders, but rather as natural forms of human variability.[2] Almost everyone in the United States deviates from John Wayne/Marilyn Monroe gender norms in some way or another, and those who do often face difficulties because of it. In the broadest sense of the term, gay men, lesbians, and everyone who challenges sexual, sartorial, behavioral, or occupational norms can be said to be to some extent transgendered (cf Signorile, 1996).

The transgender model changed the locus of pathology; if there is pathology, it might more properly be attributed to the society rather than the gender-variant individual. Those who are most visibly different are at risk for discrimination, hostility, and violence from an intolerant culture, and often from their schools, churches, police and other government officials, and even family members (Wilchins et al., 1997; see also the Remembering Our Dead website at www.gender.org/remember). Because of discrimination, many transgendered people are not able to get jobs, or, if they have them, keep them (Green and Brinkin, 1994). Marginalization can force occupational and other life choices with dire consequences for health and safety–for instance, some transgendered and transsexual women turn to sex work because they are unable to get or keep jobs due to discrimination and because there is a steady demand for transgendered sex workers. When one is faced with homelessness, denied even the most menial of jobs, sex work can sometimes provide an alternative way to pay the rent.[3]

The transgender model holds that this societal mistreatment can result in psychological difficulties, including shame and guilt and resulting self-destructive behaviors, including abuse of alcohol and other drugs, eating disorders, and self-injurious behavior; dissociative conditions; personality and behavior disorders; and mood disturbances. Accounts under the older transsexual model tended to assume such problems were symptoms of or co-existent with the "syndrome" of transsexualism, discounting or more often never even considering that they might be reactions to societal discrimination and abuse.

At first discussed only in the pages of community newsletters and magazines, the transgender model quickly found acceptance in gay and lesbian and academic circles. By the mid-1990s, the term was appearing widely in newspapers, magazines and books. A new generation of helping professionals was on the scene, questioning the orthodoxies of the transsexual model (Israel and Tarver, 1998). The model was also proving useful in promoting political, legal, and social acceptance of gender-variant people (Currah, Minter, and Green, 2000).

The transgender model appeals to many who had hesitated to call themselves transsexuals or crossdressers, including gay men and lesbians who recognize their gender variance (Signorile, 1996). The gay and lesbian community, which has had a longstanding love-hate relationship with transgendered people (Brewster, 1969; Denny, 1994), has become more welcoming, and transgender has been added to the name or mission statements of even the most recalcitrant GLB organizations (Human Rights Campaign, 2001). The model also appeals to academics, and the name transgender has been added to the titles of texts and conferences.

DISADVANTAGES OF THE TRANSGENDER MODEL

The transgender model weakens some arguments which have been successfully used to justify hormonal therapy and sex reassignment surgery. If transsexuals and other transgendered persons are not mentally ill, there is no psychiatric justification for hormonal therapy and SRS. If these technologies are not being used to provide relief for a psychiatric condition, they can be viewed as cosmetic or even frivolous in nature.

It should be noted, however, that the suffering of transsexuals is real enough, and the dissatisfaction of transsexuals with their bodies and gender of assignment has been well documented from Benjamin (1966) to present. Dozens of studies have shown sex reassignment to be effective in both male-to-female and female-to-male transsexuals (see Blanchard and Sheridan, 1990). The lone study showing "no objective advantage" to male-to-female sex reassignment (Meyer and Reter, 1979) was seriously methodologically flawed (Blanchard and Sheridan, 1990) and possibly fraudulent (Ogas, 1994).

The transgender model tends to render transsexuals invisible. While many transgendered people are comfortable fitting somewhere in the space between the two commonly acknowledged genders, transsexuals have no doubts about the gender to which they belong. They unambiguously identify with the non-natal gender. They are not necessarily comfortable in the middle spaces, and many of them find little in common with transgenderists and crossdressers and others of ambiguous gender. Transsexuals often claim they are pressured to take "the middle road" by peers and helping professionals, and may be ridiculed because of their identities as members of the non-natal sex.

This has resulted in an ideological division within the transgender community with special implications for legal protections: should nondiscrimination and hate-crime protections be extended only to those who change sex, or to those with ambiguous or alternating gender presentations?

The transgender model also threatens some existing legal protections. If a political entity offers protection from discrimination based on a perceived disability (transsexualism), what happens when that disability is destabilized? Transgender civil rights activists have asked this and similar questions. While protections based on nondiscrimination may prove to be more long-lasting, some activists believe it is beneficial to pursue legal protections on the basis of disability (see MacKenzie and Nangeroni, 2002).

THE EFFECT OF THE TRANSGENDER MODEL

Opponents of sex reassignment have been troubled by the apparent increase in the numbers of men and women who have sought and obtained sex reassignment in recent years (see McHugh, 1992). There are no national statistics on sex reassignment procedures, but certainly more and more transsexuals and other transgendered people seem to coming forward, as evidenced by increased attendance at conferences and support groups. There are a number of possible reasons for this. First, the transgender model lets gender-variant men and women view themselves as healthy and can relieve their burden of guilt and shame, helping them to come out rather than remain invisible to demographers (Denny, 1997). Second, the model appeals to nontranssexual gender-variant people. Many individuals who formerly identified as gay or lesbian, and especially genderqueer youth find it appealing.

The transgender model doesn't require the individual to be attractive or to pass as a member of the other gender and makes no restrictions based on sexual orientation, marital status, or occupation–nor does it require appearance and dress that is sterotypically male or female. Androgyny is not only acceptable, but often seen as desirable (Boswell, 1991).

In the transgender model, access to feminizing or masculinizing medical treatment is not limited to only those who seek treatment at formal gender programs; the various technologies of sex reassignment, previously available only to a few individuals after a rigorous screening process, are now available to almost anyone who desires it. Those who desire to change their bodies are not forced into a pre-arranged course that inevitably culminates in sex reassignment surgery. They can pick and choose among medical technologies, altering their bodies no more or no less than they need or wish.

The transgender model has opened a middle ground that was not possible under the model it replaced. Before about 1990, transgendered persons were expected to declare themselves to be crossdressers, who were not expected to seek sex reassignment; or transsexuals, who *were* expected to and who came under pressure from peers when they didn't (see Bolin, 1988). This situation had changed dramatically by the mid-1990s, when the same researcher found that individuals were encouraged to interpret and express their gender variance in individual ways (Bolin, 1994). Gender-variant people now self-identify in often idiosyncratic ways, many of which do not lead to hormonal therapy and SRS. Respondents to a survey by Denny and Roberts (1997) used more than 40 terms when describing themselves. Cromwell, Green and Denny's (2001) findings were similar.

The transgender model highlights some of the culturally bound assumptions of early critics of transsexualism and sex reassignment, and in so doing renders them obsolete or ineffective. For instance, if there is no mental illness, sex reassignment cannot be viewed as collaboration with mental illness (Wiedeman, 1953); since many transgendered people deliberately blend gender (Devor, 1989) and post-transition transsexuals nowadays tend to dress and look much like any other group of men and women (Bolin, 1994), transsexuals can no longer be accused of having and expressing stereotyped notions of manhood and womanhood (Raymond, 1979), for they are no longer expected by medical professionals to dress and behave in a stereotypic manner. The older literature must also be re-examined in light of the social pressures now known to be inherent in the treatment setting, particularly characterizations such as the following:

> [Transsexuals as a class] were depressed, isolated, withdrawn, schizoid individuals with profound dependency conflicts. Furthermore, they were immature, narcissistic, egocentric and potentially explosive, while their attempts to obtain [professional assistance] were demanding, manipulative, controlling, coercive, and paranoid. (Lothstein, 1979, quoted in Stone, 1991)

A modern reading raises questions as to whether the behavior characterized by Lothstein above was actually an artifact of the treatment setting.

While it is not without disadvantages, the transgender model has allowed theoretical constructions which were not possible under the older model. The transsexual model held, for instance, that there is but one type of female gender variance (see Pauly, 1992, for a discussion). Devor's (1993) data challenged this orthodoxy, and in 1997 she presented a multifactorial model of female gender variance. Without the overarching framework of the transgender model, Devor's model might never have been developed.[4]

IMPLICATIONS FOR PSYCHIATRY

The transgender model, now ten years old, has had a significant effect on interactions between transgendered persons and mental health professionals. The expectations of both caregivers and clients, and the therapy hour itself, have been affected. There is a world of difference when both the therapist and the patient believe the patient to be mentally ill and in crisis, and when both the therapist and the client believe the client to be healthy and self-actualized and contemplating a life-altering decision. There is, moreover, considerable difference between the mutual belief that the purpose of therapy is to determine whether the patient is or is not a candidate for sex reassignment and the mutual belief that the purpose of therapy is to help the client make sense of and life plans about his or her feelings about gender. In other words, even if one is transsexual, one is not required or expected to alter one's body and change gender roles–although that is certainly an option. Whether for religious reasons, out of consideration for family, or because of economic considerations, many of today's transsexuals remain in whole or in part in their original gender roles.

Today's client is likely to be educated about transgender issues, to know his or her options, and to have a broad-based support system. The therapist can and should provide factual information, help the client understand the available options, and make necessary referrals. This can prove difficult to a therapist unfamiliar with the transgender model. To the uninitiated, contemporary self-definitions may be bewildering, and the therapist may be unwilling to authorize medical procedures for a client who does not fit the "all-or-none" model of transsexualism. Similarly, a client who interprets his or her experience by way of the transsexual model may be unaware of or unwilling to acknowledge options other than sex reassignment culminating in genital surgery.

Psychiatrists and other caregivers should be careful not to confuse their personal beliefs about gender with the clinical needs of the patients they are treating. Therapists should know that despite nonsurgical lifestyle options now open to transgendered people, transsexuals tend to view SRS as the treatment of choice.[5]

Gender programs in the U.S. now offer support to all transgendered people and educate their clients about non-surgical alternatives; the Program in Human Sexuality took an early lead in this (Bockting and Coleman, 1992a; Bockting, 1997). New treatment models have been developed, in particular the transgender model used at the University of Minnesota, a well-patient model at the Comprehensive Gender Services Program of the University of Michigan Health System (Cole, 1997; Samons, 1998), and a community empowerment model used by the Gender Identity Project at the Gay and Lesbian Community Services Center of New York (Warren, Blumenstein and Walker, 1998).

The treatment literature has also come under the influence of the transgender model. Of note are works by Cole et al. (2000), Bockting and Coleman (1992b), Denny (1998), and Israel and Tarver (1998), all of whom use terminology quite different from the earlier literature. Texts by authors who have been influenced by the transgender model (Brown and Rounsley, 1996; Ettner, 1996, 1999) are easily contrasted to works by authors who have not (Ramsey, 1996; Lothstein, 1983).

A paradigm change is a scientific revolution of sorts (Kuhn, 1962), and those who are fortunate enough to be around when one occurs stand to learn a grand deal. Far from upsetting the apple cart, the rise of the transgender model has provided new opportunities for researchers and clinicians and transsexuals alike.

NOTES

1. Usually referred by the acronym, HBIGDA. Formed in the late 1960s and named after the physician who defined the syndrome of transsexualism, HBIGDA is a professional organization for those who are associated in a professional capacity with gender-variant people. HBIGDA's Standards of Care, first published in 1979, are revised periodically. For its first 20 years, HBIGDA was concerned exclusively with transsexualism, but by the late 1990s had broadened its focus to encompass nontranssexual transgendered people. The International Journal of Transgenderism is available online at www.symposion.com/ijt.

2. History and anthropological studies seem to support this; gender-variant roles are documented in many tribal societies, and Western culture has hundreds of examples of historical figures whose behavior and dress varied greatly from the norms of the place and time (see especially Bullough and Bullough, 1993; Herdt, 1994; Taylor, 1996).

3. Transgendered and transsexual sex workers are at high risk for HIV/AIDS. Studies in several cities have revealed high levels of HIV seropositivity among transgendered sex workers (see Xavier, 2001a, for a review and Xavier, 2001b, for a discussion of implications for health care policy).

4. Female-to-male transsexuals, once considered rare (Pauly, 1969), and rendered virtually invisible under the transsexual model (see Cromwell, 1999 for a discussion), have become more visible under the transgender model (Green and Wilchins, 1996) and have garnered much press (Bloom, 1994).

5. The transgender model has opened new possibilities for nontranssexual gender-variant people, but transsexuals aren't necessarily interested in new interpretations of manhood and womanhood or exploring a gender middle-ground. They don't wish for more freedom in their natal sex roles, but to be members of the other sex.

REFERENCES

American Psychiatric Association (1980), *Diagnostic and Statistical Manual of Mental Disorders, 3rd Ed. Washington, DC: American Psychiatric Association.*

_____ (1994), *Diagnostic and Statistical Manual of Mental Disorders, 4th Ed.* Washington, DC: American Psychiatric Association.

Baastrup, P.C. (1966), Transvestism–A psychiatric symptom. World Congress of Psychiatry IV. *Excerpta Medica International Congress Series*, 117:109.

Benjamin, H. (1966), *The Transsexual Phenomenon: A Scientific Report on Transsexualism and Sex Conversion in the Human Male and Female.* New York: Julian Press.

_____ (1969), Introduction. In: *Transsexualism and Sex Reassignment*, eds. R. Green & J. Money. Baltimore: The Johns Hopkins University Press, pp. 1-10.

Blanchard, R. & Sheridan, P.M. (1990), Gender reorientation and psychosocial adjustment. In: *Clinical Management of Gender Identity Disorders in Children and Adults,* eds. R. Blanchard & B. Steiner. Washington, DC: American Psychiatric Press, pp. 159-189.

Bloom, A. (1994), The body lies. *The New Yorker*, pp. 38-49, July 17.

Blumer, D. (1969), Transsexualism, sexual dysfunction, and temporal lobe disorder. In: *Transsexualism and Sex Reassignment*, eds. R. Green & J. Money. Baltimore: The Johns Hopkins University Press, pp. 213-219.

Bockting, W.O. (1997), Transgender coming out: Implications for the clinical management of gender dysphoria. In: *Gender Blending*, eds. B. Bullough, V.L. Bullough & J. Elias. Amherst, NY: Prometheus Press, pp. 48-52.

_____ & Coleman, E. (1992a), A comprehensive approach to the treatment of gender dysphoria. In: *Gender Dysphoria: Interdisciplinary Approaches to Clinical Management*, eds. W. Bockting & E. Coleman. New York: Haworth Press, pp. 131-155.

_____ & Coleman, E., eds. (1992b), *Gender Dysphoria: Interdisciplinary Approaches in Clinical Management*. New York: The Haworth Press.

Bolin, A.E. (1988), *In Search of Eve: Transsexual Rites of Passage*. South Hadley, MA: Bergin & Garvey Publishers, Inc.

_____ (1994), Transcending and transgendering: Male-to-female transsexuals, dichotomy, and diversity. In: *Third Sex, Third Gender: Essays from Anthropology and Social History*, ed. G. Herdt. New York: Zone Publishing, pp. 447-485.

Bornstein, K. (1994), *Gender Outlaw: On Men, Women, and the Rest of Us*. New York: Routledge.

Boswell, H. (1991), The transgender alternative. *Chrysalis Quart.*, 1:29-31.

Brewster, L. (1969), Editorial. *Drag*, 1:1.

Brown, M. & Rounsley, C.A. (1996), *True Selves: Understanding Transsexualism for Family, Friends, Coworkers, and Helping Professionals*. San Francisco: Jossey-Bass Publishers.

Bullough, V.L. & Bullough, B. (1993), *Cross-Dressing, Sex, and Gender*. Philadelphia: University of Pennsylvania Press.

Cole, S.S. (1997), The University of Michigan Comprehensive Gender Services Program. Paper presented at the Second International Congress on Sex and Gender Issues, King of Prussia, PA, 19-22 June, 1997.

Cromwell, J. (1999), *Transmen & FTMs: Identities, Bodies, Genders, and Sexualities*. Urbana: University of Illinois Press.

_____, Green, J. & Denny, D. (2001), The language of gender variance. Paper presented at XVII HBIGDA International Symposium on Gender Dysphoria, Galveston, TX, 31 October-4 November.

Currah, P., Minter, S. & Green, J. (2000), *Transgender Equality: A Handbook for Activists and Policymakers*. Washington, DC: National Gay and Lesbian Task Force.

Denny, D. (1992), The politics of diagnosis and a diagnosis of politics: The university-affiliated gender clinics, and how they failed to meet the needs of transsexual people. *Chrysalis Quart.*, 1:9-20.

_____ (1994), You're strange and we're wonderful: The gay/lesbian and transgender communities. In: *Bound by Diversity: Essays, Prose, Photography, and Poetry by Members of the Lesbian, Bisexual, Gay, and Transgender Communities*, ed. J. Sears. Columbia, SC: Sebastian Press.

_____ (1995), The paradigm shift is here! *AEGIS News*, 1:4-5.

_____ (1997), Transgender: Some historical, cross-cultural, and modern-day models and methods of coping & treatment. In: *Gender Blending,* eds. B. Bullough, V.A. Bullough & J. Elias. Amherst, NY: Prometheus Books, pp. 33-47.

_____, ed. (1998), *Current Concepts in Transgender Identity*. New York: Garland Publishers.

_____ & Roberts, J. (1997), Results of a survey of consumer attitudes about the HBIGDA Standards of Care. In: *Gender Blending,* eds. B. Bullough, V.A. Bullough & J. Elias. Amherst, NY: Prometheus Books, pp. 320-336.

Devor, H. (1989), *Gender Blending: Confronting the Limits of Duality*. Bloomington: Indiana University Press.

_____ (1993), Sexual orientation, identities, attractions, and practices of female-to-male transsexuals. *J. of Sex Res.*, 30:303-315.

_____ (1997), A social context for gender dysphoria. Paper presented at the XV Harry Benjamin International Gender Dysphoria Association Symposium: The State of Our Art and the State of Our Science, Vancouver, British Columbia, Canada, 10-13 September, 1997.

Ettner, R. (1996), *Confessions of a Gender Defender: A Psychologist's Reflections on Life Among the Transgendered*. Evanston, IL: Chicago Spectrum Press.

_____ (1999), *Gender Loving Care: A Guide to Counseling Gender-Variant Clients*. New York: W.W. Norton.

Green, J. & Brinkin, L. (1994), *Investigation Into Discrimination Against Transgendered People*. San Francisco, CA: Human Rights Commission, City and County of San Francisco.

_____ & Wilchins, R.A. (1996), New men on the horizon. *FTM Internat. Newslet.*, 33, January.

Green, R. (1969), Conclusion. In: *Transsexualism and Sex Reassignment*, eds. R. Green & J. Money. Baltimore: The Johns Hopkins University Press, pp. 467-473.

_____ & Money, J., eds. (1969), *Transsexualism and Sex Reassignment*. Baltimore: The Johns Hopkins University Press.

Hamburger, C. (1953), The desire for change of sex as shown by personal letters from 465 men and women. *Acta Endocrinologica*, 14:361-375.

Herdt, G. ed. (1994), *Third Sex, Third Gender: Essays from Anthropology and Social History*. New York: Zone Books.

Hoenig, J. (1985), Etiology of transsexualism. In: *Gender Dysphoria: Development, Research, Management*, ed. B. Steiner. New York: Plenum Press, pp. 33-73.

Human Rights Campaign. (2001), Speaking about gender expression and identity (Press release). Washington, DC: Human Rights Campaign, March 23.

Israel, G. & Tarver, D. (1998), *Transgender Care: Recommended Guidelines, Practical Information, and Personal Accounts*. Philadelphia, PA: Temple University Press.

Kessler, S.J. & McKenna, W. (1978), *Gender: An Ethnomethodological Approach*. New York: John Wiley & Sons. Reprinted in 1985 by The University of Chicago Press.

Kuhn, T.S. (1962), *The Structure of Scientific Revolutions*. Chicago: The University of Chicago.

Lothstein, L.M. (1979), The aging gender dysphoria (transsexual) patient. *Arch. Sex. Behav.*, 8:431-444.

_____ (1983), *Female-to-Male Transsexualism: Historical, Clinical and Theoretical Issues*. Boston: Routledge & Kegan Paul.

MacKenzie, G. & Nangeroni, N. (2002), Profile: Jennifer Levi: Attorney for gender justice. *Transgender Tapestry*, 1:28-33.

McHugh, P. (1992), Psychiatric misadventures. *Amer. Scholar*, 61:497-510.

Meyer, J.K. & Reter, D. (1979), Sex reassignment: Follow-up. *Arch. Gen. Psychiat.*, 36:1010-1015.

Newman, L.E. & Stoller, R.J. (1974), Nontranssexual men who seek sex reassignment. *Amer. J. Psychiat.*, 131:437-441.

Ogas, O. (1994), Spare parts: New information reignites a controversy surrounding the Hopkins gender identity clinic. *City Paper* (Baltimore), 18:cover, 10-15, March 9.

Ostow, M. (1953), Transvestism (Letter to the editor). *JAMA*, 152:1553.

Pauly, I.B. (1969), Adult manifestations of male transsexualism. In: *Transsexualism and Sex Reassignment*, eds. R. Green & J. Money. Baltimore: The Johns Hopkins University Press, pp. 37-87.

_____(1992), Review of L. Sullivan, *From Female to Male: The Life of Jack Bee Garland. Arch. Sex. Behav.*, 21:201-204.

Petersen, M.A. & Dickey, R. (1995), Surgical sex reassignment: A comparative survey of international centers. *Arch. Sex. Behav.*, 24:135-156.

Prince, C.V. (1973), Sex vs. gender. In: *Proceedings of the Second International Symposium on Gender Dysphoria Syndrome*, eds. D. Laub & P. Gandy. Palo Alto, CA: Stanford University Medical Center, pp. 20-24.

Ramsey, J. (1996), *Transsexuals: Candid Answers to Private Questions*. Freedom, CA: The Crossing Press.

Raymond, J. (1979), *The Transsexual Empire: The Making of the She-Male*. Boston: Beacon Press. Reissued in 1994 by Teacher's College Press, New York.

Rothblatt, M. (1994), *The Apartheid of Sex: A Manifesto on the Freedom of Gender*. New York: Crown Publishers.

Samons, S. (1998), Mental health preventive/well-care for the M > F transgendered client. Presented at Joint Annual Meeting, The Society for the Scientific Study of Sexuality and the American Association of Sex Educators, Counselors & Therapists, 11-15 November, 1998, Los Angeles, CA.

Signorile, M. (1996), Transgender nation. *Out*: June, last page.

Socarides, C.W. (1969), The desire for sexual transformation: A psychiatric evaluation of transsexualism. *Amer. J. Psychiat.*, 125:1419-1425.

Spensley, J. & Barter, J.T. (1971), The adolescent transvestite on a psychiatric service: Family patterns. *J. Sex. Behav.*, 1:347-356.

Stone, A.R. (as Sandy Stone) (1991), The *empire* strikes back: A posttranssexual manifesto. In: *Body Guards: The Cultural Politics of Gender Ambiguity*, eds. J. Epstein & K. Straub. New York: Routledge, pp. 280-304.

Stone, C.B. (1977), Psychiatric screening for transsexual surgery. *Psychosomatics*, 18:25-27.

Taylor, T. (1996), *The Prehistory of Sex: Four Million Years of Human Sexual Culture*. New York: Bantam Books.

Warren, B.E., Blumenstein, R. & Walker, L. (1998), Appendix: The empowerment of a community. In: *Current Concepts in Transgender Identity*, ed. D. Denny. New York: Garland Publishing, pp. 427-430.

Wiedeman, G.H. (1953), Letter to the editor. *JAMA*, 152:1167.

Wilchins, R.A., Lombardi, L., Priesing, D. & Malouf, D. (1997), *Genderpac First National Survey of Transgender Violence.* New York: Genderpac.

Xavier, J.M. (2001a), HIV/AIDS in transgender populations. *Psychology & Aids Exchange* (American Psychological Association), 1:4,16-20, Summer.

_____ (2001b), Transgendered people and public health policy. *Psychology & Aids Exchange* (American Psychological Association), 1:4,17,19-20,22, Summer.

Witnessing and Mirroring:
A Fourteen Stage Model
of Transsexual Identity Formation

Aaron H. Devor, PhD

SUMMARY. Coming to recognize oneself as transsexual involves a number of stages of exploration and analysis on both an interpersonal and intrapersonal level over the course of many years. A model encompassing fourteen possible stages is proposed: (1) Abiding Anxiety, (2) Identity Confusion About Originally Assigned Gender and Sex, (3) Identity Comparisons About Originally Assigned Gender and Sex, (4) Discovery of Transsexualism, (5) Identity Confusion About Transsexualism, (6) Identity Comparisons About Transsexualism, (7) Tolerance of Transsexual Identity, (8) Delay Before Acceptance of Transsexual Identity, (9) Acceptance of Transsexualism Identity, (10) Delay Before Transition, (11) Transition, (12) Acceptance of Post-Transition Gender and Sex Identities, (13) Integration, and (14) Pride. *[Article copies available for a fee from The Haworth Document Delivery Service: 1-800-HAWORTH. E-mail address: <docdelivery@haworthpress.com> Website: <http://www. HaworthPress.com> © 2004 by The Haworth Press, Inc. All rights reserved.]*

Aaron H. Devor is Dean of Graduate Studies, and Professor in the Sociology Department, University of Victoria. He is the author of *Gender Blending: Confronting the Limits of Duality*, and *FTM: Female-to-Male Transsexuals in Society*.

Address correspondence to: Aaron H. Devor, PhD, Sociology Department, University of Victoria, Box 3050, Victoria, BC V8W 3P5, Canada (E-mail: ahdevor@uvic.ca).

[Haworth co-indexing entry note]: "Witnessing and Mirroring: A Fourteen Stage Model of Transsexual Identity Formation." Devor, Aaron H. Co-published simultaneously in *Journal of Gay & Lesbian Psychotherapy* (The Haworth Medical Press, an imprint of The Haworth Press, Inc.) Vol. 8, No. 1/2, 2004, pp. 41-67; and: *Transgender Subjectivities: A Clinician's Guide* (ed: Ubaldo Leli, and Jack Drescher) The Haworth Medical Press, an imprint of The Haworth Press, Inc., 2004, pp. 41-67. Single or multiple copies of this article are available for a fee from The Haworth Document Delivery Service [1-800-HAWORTH, 9:00 a.m. - 5:00 p.m. (EST). E-mail address: docdelivery@haworthpress.com].

KEYWORDS. Anxiety, female-to-male, FTM, identity formation, male-to-female, mirroring, MTF, sex reassignment, sociology, transgender, transsexual, witnessing

INTRODUCTION

Most transsexed people and most of the professionals who work with them believe that ultimately a biological basis for transsexualism will be found. Nevertheless, no matter how much of our lives may be ruled by biological considerations, all people live within social environments which give meanings to the realities of their bodies and of their psyches. Over the course of our lifetimes, each of us biological organisms must learn how to understand ourselves as we grow and adapt to a shifting and changing world.

What is proposed here is a fourteen-stage model of transsexual identity formation (Table 1). This model is built upon a model of homosexual identity formation developed by Cass (1979, 1984, 1990) and upon Ebaugh's (1988) work about role exit. Although the focus here will be transsexed people, this paper will also attempt to explain some of the ways in which the model might apply for other transgendered people.

This model is based on the author's twenty years of sociological field research, personal experience, social and professional interactions with a wide range of transgendered persons–the majority of whom have self-identified as female-to-male transsexed or transgendered (Devor, 1987, 1989, 1993, 1994, 1997a, 1997b, 1997c; Kendal, Devor and Strapko, 1997; Meyer et al., 2001). The data base for these propositions includes personal experience and contacts with hundreds of transsexed and transgendered people in settings such as face-to-face in-depth structured interviews, each lasting several hours, extended private consultations, innumerable heart-to-heart conversations in private settings, extended visits in one another's homes, private house parties, meetings at community and professional conferences, dinners, lunches, walks on the beach, and hard-working task-oriented committees of professional organizations; in other words, a wide variety of non-clinical settings.

In reviewing this model it is important to bear in mind that it cannot possibly apply to all individuals in the same way. Each person is unique. Each person experiences their world in their own idiosyncratic ways. Some people may never experience some of these stages. Some people may pass through some stages more quickly and others more slowly. Whereas some people may move through these stages in their own particular order, some people may repeat some stages several times, while the model may be totally inapplicable to others.

TABLE 1

Stages of Transsexual or Transgender Identity Formation		
Stage	Some Characteristics	Some Actions
1) Abiding Anxiety	Unfocussed gender and sex discomfort.	Preference for other gender activities and companionship.
2) Identity Confusion About Originally Assigned Gender and Sex	First doubts about suitability of originally assigned gender and sex.	Reactive gender and sex conforming activities.
3) Identity Comparisons About Originally Assigned Gender and Sex	Seeking and weighing alternative gender identities.	Experimenting with alternative gender consistent identities.
4) Discovery of Transsexualism or Transgenderism	Learning that transsexualism or transgenderism exists.	Accidental contact with information about transsexualism or transgenderism
5) Identity Confusion About Transsexualism or Transgenderism	First doubts about the authenticity of own transsexualism or transgenderism.	Seeking more information about transsexualism or transgenderism.
6) Identity Comparisons About Transsexualism or Transgenderism	Testing transsexual or transgender identity using transsexual or transgender reference group.	Start to disindentify with originally assigned sex and gender. Start to identify as transsexed or transgender.
7) Tolerance of Transsexual or Transgender Identity	Identify as probably transsexual or transgender.	Increasingly disidentify as originally assigned gender and sex.
8) Delay Before Acceptance of Transsexual or Transgender Identity	Waiting for changed circumstances. Looking for confirmation of transsexual or transgender identity.	Seeking more information about transsexualism or transgenderism. Reality testing in intimate relationships and against further information about transsexualism or transgenderism.
9) Acceptance of Transsexual or Transgender Identity	Transsexual or transgender identity established.	Tell others about transsexual or transgender identity.
10) Delay Before Transition	Transsexual identity deepens. Final disidentity as original gender and sex. Anticipatory socialization.	Learning how to do transition. Saving money. Organizing support systems.
11) Transition	Changing genders and sexes.	Gender and sex reassignments.
12) Acceptance of Post-Transition Gender and Sex Identities	Post-transition identity established.	Successful post-transition living.
13) Integration	Transsexuality mostly invisible.	Stigma management. Identity integration.
14) Pride	Openly transsexed.	Transsexual advocacy.

It is also important to remember that any person may enter into a process which resembles the one outlined here but may conclude that the best way for them to live their lives is to go no further than any particular stage. Just because an individual may seem to be following the trajectory described herein does not mean that they will end up making any particular choice for any particular outcome. This model is only intended to provide some insights into a commonly followed path. It is by no means the only path, nor will all who appear to be following it come to the same conclusions.

A SOCIAL CONTEXT

In a social psychological sense, the phenomena which are recognized as transsexualism only make sense within a social context which is predicated upon a number of primary assumptions about the nature of sex and gender. What is outlined here pertains to contemporary mainstream Euro-American values. Social groups who do not share these assumptions make sense of gender variations in their own culturally specific ways.

In order for transsexualism to be a meaningful concept, widely accepted social values must dictate that clearly distinct categories of gender and sex exist independently of social will. Furthermore, it must be accepted that genders and sexes are ultimately verifiable only on the basis of specific physical attributes. These societal beliefs, however, are themselves social products of particular cultures under particular historical conditions (Fausto-Sterling, 2000; Laqueur, 1990). Thus, transsexualism only makes sense within the context of a society in which there exists a nearly universally accepted way of understanding gender which teaches people to function as if certain ideological presumptions were elemental truths rather than the products of particular social arrangements.

Such a way of understanding gender presumes that there are two and only two biological sexes, male and female, and that under "normal" circumstances persons' sexes are unchanging and can be definitively determined from a visual inspection of their genitalia. Similar underlying assumptions about gender must also be accepted for transsexualism to make sense. That is to say that we must believe that there are only two social genders, men/boys and women/girls, and that under "normal" circumstances persons' gender classifications are unchanging and can be determined by casual visual inspection of persons in everyday social situations. Furthermore, it must be assumed that sex and gender are inextricably linked in a fixed and biologically natural way: all males are men/boys and all females are women/girls. In this schema there are no socially-acceptable intermediate sexes, no socially-acceptable intermediate genders. Within this world view, such gender or sex indeterminacy will only make social sense within a context of it being an illness which must be corrected as soon as possible.

Although primary sex characteristics have the role of being the only legitimate markers of sex status in everyday life, genitalia are rarely directly displayed or discussed. Rather, gender styles of femininity and masculinity are the media of most social exchange. As such, gender styles indicate genders and genders act as markers of sexes. Persons who seamlessly perform particular gender styles are attributed by others with being the corresponding gender and sex. Thus, although the common assumption is that genders are the result of people being particular sexes, people functionally read gender styles, genders, and sexes in the reverse order. That is to say that in everyday life, we actually read gender on the basis of gender styles, not on the basis of sexes. In other words, under most circumstances, people are assumed to be either male or female, men or women, on the basis of social characteristics, mannerisms, and personality traits. Such attributions are usually made automatically and with little or no conscious thought and are accompanied by the assumption that genders and sexes are permanent and unchangeable.

Therefore, persons who wish to be taken as a particular gender and sex have few options open to them. They may successfully perform as the gender of their choice and rely on people's assumptions to attribute them with the desired sex as well. However, the success of such performances can be entirely unseated by the disclosure of sex characteristics which do not match the gender being presented. Therefore, no matter how effective persons' performances of their genders may be, the most reliable option open to them is to unequivocally substantiate their claim to being a particular gender by also possessing the sex characteristics socially designated as appropriate. In order for persons to socially legitimate their gender identity claims, they must ultimately have bodies which match their gender claims in socially expected ways.

The model presented here traces one of the most common pathways used by people in the process of coming to understand that they are transsexed. It outlines how they first come to feel that they do not belong as members of their originally assigned sex and gender and later to understand themselves as members of another gender and sex. It also describes how they learn to think of themselves as transsexed in order to make sense of the apparent contradiction of being born to one sex and gender while knowing themselves to belong as another (Tully, 1992).

WITNESSING AND MIRRORING

There are two overarching themes which run throughout the entire process of transsexual identity formation which, indeed, run though the lives of many people as they search for self-understanding. Each of us are social beings and as such we live in a sea of other humans with whom we interact during most of the waking hours of our lives. Even when we are not in contact with others, we devote a tremendous amount of our psychic energies to being psychologically engaged with others. It would therefore be difficult to underestimate the powerful effects that the opinions of others have on each of us.

Each of us has a deep need to be witnessed by others for whom we are. Each of us wants to see ourselves mirrored in others' eyes as we see ourselves. These interactive processes, witnessing and mirroring, are part of everyone's lives. When they work well, we feel validated and confirmed–our sense of self is reinforced (Poland, 2000). When the messages which one receives back from others do not match how one feels inside, various kinds of psychological distress and maladaptive behaviors can result. When the situation is especially severe it can lead to psychotic and/or suicidal behaviors.

Although they are closely related in that they both serve a purpose of validation of self, witnessing and mirroring involve somewhat different processes, different personnel, and different kinds of feedback. Each of us is defined both by who we are and by who we are not. The effectiveness of witnesses, in part, derives from the fact that they are not like oneself and can look at us from outside of our categories of self-definition. Witnesses can be presumed to have some distance and therefore to have some perspective and objectivity about their observations. When dispassionate witnesses provide appraisals which conform to one's own sense of self, it leaves one with a feeling of having been accurately seen by others who can be assumed to be impartial. Thus, validations offered by non-transgendered friends, loved ones, co-workers, and interested professionals of the gender and sex identities of transgendered people can serve as a powerful reinforcer of transgendered identities. Conversely, when what a whole society witnesses clashes with persons' self-images, a profound alteration or destruction of that self may be appear to be the only options. Transsexualism can allow people who feel overwhelmingly unwitnessed to make sense of why others cannot see them as they see themselves. Transition allows them to make changes that enable others to witness them as they see themselves. Transsexualism thus can allow severely and chronically unwitnessed people to survive and to thrive. However, if one is only witnessed and never mirrored one can end up feeling profoundly alone in the world. One can feel as if they are the only one of their kind.

Mirroring, as I use it here, differs from Kohut's self-psychology (1984). Mirroring, in the sense that I use it here, is also about seeing oneself in the eyes of others like oneself. As well as needing to be witnessed by people who are different from ourselves, each of us also needs to be seen and validated by people who are like ourselves. We need to be seen by people who have insider knowledge of what it means to be a member of the social groups within which we identify ourselves. Each of us needs to know that people who we think are like us also see us as like them. We need to know that we are recognized and accepted by our peers. We need to know that we are not alone. For these reasons it is vitally important that transsexed and transgendered people be able to see their own feelings and experiences reflected back to them in the lives of other transsexed and transgendered people. Furthermore, the gender and sex identities of transsexed people benefit greatly from seeing that their perspectives on the world match, in key ways, with those of people who were originally assigned to the gender and sex with which they identify.

STAGE 1: ABIDING ANXIETY

The first stage of this fourteen-step model of transsexual identity formation involves a sense of abiding anxiety about one's gender and sex. This sense of not feeling right in one's social role and/or body may be traced back to one's earliest memories, or it may develop slowly over time at a later stage of life. Most commonly, transsexed people report that this sense of gender anxiety has always been with them even before they were able to say what it was that was making them uncomfortable. Eventually, it becomes clear to such individuals that the source of their anxiety lies in gender relations. It will often begin simply as a feeling of generalized discomfort around people, a sense of not fitting in or of being socially awkward. However, over time, the sense of unease becomes more clearly focused, probably because such individuals come to recognize that their preferences are for companionship and/or activities socially expected from people of another gender than the one to which they have been assigned at birth. Females prefer the activities and/or companionship of males; males prefer to be with females doing the things that females usually prefer to do. For example a 47-year-old white transman home healthcare worker remembered it like this:

> I didn't have friends. I just wasn't comfortable with people. Casual acquaintances, but I did not have friends. I'd see them at school and yes we would speak if we saw each other but that was it. It was just too uncomfortable. With the girls, it was simply I was not interested in the same things. I don't think I gave people a chance. I know that all through my life people have had a problem relating to me. There was a discomfort and I think it went both ways. I think it was my identity. There was always something, people weren't comfortable with me.

In a highly gender dichotomized world, this is enough to make a person have trouble living comfortably as their assigned gender because others will rarely either witness or mirror them accurately. The more pronounced the mismatch between their gender preferences and society's expectations, the more pervasive will be their feelings of abiding anxiety and the greater their psychological and social difficulties will become. Over the course of many years this kind of abiding anxiety can accrete until it becomes unbearably difficult to function in society. Many people struggling with these issues turn to drugs or alcohol to relieve some of the unremitting anxiety. For some people, the distress can become so acute that suicide seems to be the only option.

STAGE 2: IDENTITY CONFUSION
ABOUT ORIGINALLY ASSIGNED GENDER AND SEX

One response to the realization that one does not fit in well with others of their gender, when one cannot find others like themselves to mirror them, is to question whether one really is supposed to be their assigned gender or sex at all. Children may become quite completely convinced that they are in the wrong gender and the wrong sex and may proclaim loudly to others that they are actually members of the preferred gender and sex. However, parents, teachers, and peers will routinely do everything in their power to disabuse them of such ideas because they witness them as belonging in their originally assigned gender and sex. This kind of social and psychological pressure to conformity is usually enough to cause children to either temporarily abandon or hide these kinds of gender thoughts from others and/or from themselves (Zucker and Bradley, 1995). Although they may still believe that they really are or should be another sex and gender, many children simply stop talking about it, fantasize a different future for themselves and wait for puberty to bring about the changes that they believe are their due. When puberty arrives and their bodies do not turn into the ones they had imagined for themselves, many transgendered people fall into severe depression, substance abuse, and suicidality. A 36-year-old white transit manager recalled these experiences:

> Ever since I've been twelve I've felt like I was in the wrong body. It was like "Oh, this isn't going to happen." So I think from [puberty] on I was pretty unhappy about my gender, I felt restricted in my activities. It just didn't feel comfortable for me at all. So it was like to me it didn't make any sense at all that I was the way I was physically. It didn't click. Well, from twelve to eighteen I was basically drinking all during that period. In fact, I remember going to school, most of the time I'd drink a couple of shots of vodka and smoke a little bit of pot before I even walked across the street. So basically I was just taking drugs.

Adolescents and adults may also respond to abiding gender anxieties by feeling confusion about the appropriateness of their originally assigned gender/sex. Because they will have learned and internalized more completely the social rules of gender, they are even less likely to speak of their gender confusion publicly. Teens and adults will understand that there will most probably be a great deal of stigma attached to any proclamations about doubts that they may be having about the correctness of their originally assigned gender or their originally assigned sex. They will know the social rules which insist that one's sex unequivocally determines one's gender. They will understand that to claim otherwise is to invite others to think of them as crazy.

At any age, the social and psychological realities will at first push most individuals into hiding. Children, adolescents, and adults will often react to these feelings of identity confusion by trying harder to make themselves conform more exactly to social expectations about appropriately gendered behaviors. Most commonly they will react to their gender identity confusion with an honest attempt to look and act as persons assigned to their sex are supposed to look and act, even if on the inside that is not how they feel. One 41-year-old white unemployed transman recalled:

> As I did reach adolescence where certain things were kind of required of you–the dating, the things you're supposed to do as a female–I tried to do [them]. Not because I wanted to, but because I didn't want them to know that I was different. And maybe in a sense I didn't want to accept that I was different at that stage. I really wanted to be what other people wanted me to be. And I really tried to be that.

Thus it may be that even people who seem to be perfectly well adjusted to their gender roles may be harboring repressed or hidden feelings of abiding gender anxiety. This stage may be quite brief or may persist for the better part of a lifetime.

STAGE 3: IDENTITY COMPARISONS
ABOUT ORIGINALLY ASSIGNED GENDER AND SEX

Identity confusion will commonly persist and coexist with the next stage, identity comparisons. At this stage, individuals are generally accepting of the fact that the physical sex of their body has mandated their gender status and they attempt to find ways to successfully navigate between social expectations and their own needs for self-expression. During this period, individuals will try to find more comfortable ways to live as their originally-assigned gender while also expressing some of their feelings of belonging to another gender. They know what sex and gender they are and will try on alternative forms of gender expression which will allow them to better fit within the social expectations of their originally assigned gender and sex statuses.

This stage involves comparison in the sense that individuals compare their inner feelings to various types of alternative behaviors and identities that they have known others of their gender and sex to exhibit (e.g., "sensitive artiste" or "butch dyke"). If the comparisons wear well, they may adopt those ways of being and stay with them for a short while, or for the remainder of their lives. When successful, this strategy can result in individuals feeling both more witnessed and better mirrored because they can be recognized as a known type of man or woman. They can exhibit more of their inner selves for others to witness and they can find ways to share more common ground with others of their originally assigned gender and sex, thus seeing more of themselves mirrored back. If comparisons fail, individuals will keep searching for an answer to the question, "Who am I?"

Such attempts at accommodation can take many forms. For girls, the tomboy role is readily available and carries with it few disincentives. Until puberty, most girls are allowed to experiment with masculinity within the relatively comfortable confines of this socially acknowledged and accepted variant form of gender role expression. Although the tomboy role is not universally accepted, and although there are limitations on how much masculinity a girl may incorporate before arousing social ire, most of those girls who adopt the tomboy role navigate through childhood relatively psychically unscathed because such girls are able to be socially recognized and accepted *as girls* at the same time as they are able to express some of their masculinity. At puberty, however, tomboyism rapidly becomes unacceptable and those girls who do not abandon it begin to suffer from the effects of escalating social disapproval.

However, the emotional stability of girls who are too masculine for the social environments in which they live can become undermined as a result of rejections from peers and adults from a very early age. Their mental health often becomes even more precarious when they reach puberty and have to face unwelcome changes in their bodies and increased social demands for femininity.

Boys who wish to find a way to incorporate some femininity into their gendered performances have no socially acceptable format in which to present themselves. The sissy role is generally demeaned by children and adults alike. Those boys who adopt it are most often subjected to sorely psychologically and socially damaging ridicule and rejection and to abuse of all forms. Thus, feminine boys are even less likely than masculine girls to reach adolescence relatively unscathed. Sissies are extremely likely to be badly taunted and physically abused, especially by male peers and adults, leaving them feeling especially terrorized around other males and even more alienated from maleness and men.

During their adult years, people who will later come to identify themselves as transsexed or transgendered may likewise avail themselves of any of a number of techniques of identity comparison to try to determine if there is an identity within which they can comfortably live their lives in their originally assigned gender and sex.

Females may attempt to carry on as some kind of grown-up tomboy. In many cases this translates into an identity as a butch lesbian by way of the popular perception that lesbians are women who want to be men (Devor, 1997b). Feeling like men and believing that lesbians are women who want to be men, many transgendered females experiment extensively with lesbianism or bisexuality. Those females who take this course of action will often find that there are many women, and more than a few men, who witness, mirror, appreciate, and encourage their masculinity. However, at the same time masculine lesbians will, in large measure, bear the brunt of still widespread social condemnation of homosexuality. Although they find reinforcement for their masculinity in their love lives, the more masculine they are the less support and the more abuse they will suffer socially. Some heterosexually or bisexually-inclined females may also carry over their butch personas into their adult lives. Regardless of their sexual orientation, butch females will suffer from social disapproval and bear psychic scars as a result. One 33-year-old white transman artist put it this way:

> I changed my name, cut my hair short, began buying more male clothes. I lived as a male in my own eyes more, but to other people I was still a female, and I was becoming what they considered a very bizarre female. Nobody really understood it. I didn't clearly understand it myself. It was more of a subconscious manifestation of my true personality.

Similarly, males may become drawn to lifestyles which allow them a community in which to express their inherent femininity. Also having absorbed societal beliefs that all gay men are effeminate, some males may try on lives as gay or bisexual men as extensions of their sissy-boy childhoods. Some of them may be drawn to the drag scene where they will be given room to call themselves by female names, dress in women's clothing, and be appreciated for their femininity. Others may simply enact femininity in smaller more subtle ways in their everyday lives. Despite the benefits of a certain amount of witnessing and mirroring from lovers and within the restricted social environments of gay life and the drag scene, intense social disapproval of femininity in men will inevitably deeply color their experiences and leave them damaged by the scorn and discrimination to which visibly feminine men are routinely subjected.

Heterosexual males may also explore crossdressing, first in private and later more publicly, in an attempt to give expression to their inner feelings of womanliness. Usually, in the early years of the practice, such crossdressing is solitary and accompanied by sexual arousal and orgasm. Erections and ejaculations while crossdressed are often felt as concurrently satisfying, confusing, and shameful. Despite such conflicting feelings, the erections and ejaculations which accompany this kind of crossdressing can provide a concrete confirmation of maleness which can fortify one's originally assigned gender and sex identities for many years. Thus, the sexual aspect of crossdressing may allow a man to continue to feel that he is really a man while also allowing him to feel himself to be a woman. Nonetheless, crossdressing is highly stigmatized and therefore those who make use of this avenue will usually suffer significant challenges to their psychological health because of the anxieties connected with fear of exposure and the consequences of the disapproval of others.

Some people adopt a feminist critique of gender as a social construction. From this perspective, they are able to make comparisons between their own desired gender expressions and the deficiencies of standard gender roles. They may be able to find comfort in believing that the failure is not their own but rather that of a system which makes unhealthy and unobtainable gender demands on its citizens. A feminist stance may therefore allow some people to find relief in the validation of their gender non-conformity as political correctness (Devor, 1997c).

Each of these techniques may be employed so as to allow individuals to continue to have others see them and to continue to see themselves as perhaps a bit odd but still as members of their originally assigned gender and sex. To the degree that they are successful, they may remain at this stage for lengthy periods of time. Those people who define themselves as transgendered may find that they are able to make use of these options indefinitely.

STAGE 4: DISCOVERY
OF TRANSSEXUALISM OR TRANSGENDERISM

There comes a time in the life of every person who will one day identify themselves as transsexed or transgendered when they first learn that transsexualism or transgenderism exists. Some people learn of transsexualism or transgenderism at an early age. For most people this event takes place later in their lives, after many years of living with feelings of abiding anxiety, identity confusions and identity comparisons. For some people, the knowledge that transsexualism or transgenderism exists comes as a godsend which immediately crystallizes the feelings with which they have been living for many years. For many it is an "Aha!" kind of moment where everything that they have been feeling finally falls into place. Finally, they have found a mirror in which they can see themselves. Who they feel themselves to be makes sense to them for the first time. They have a name for what they feel and a possible course of action. For most people, this realization constitutes the beginning of another cycle of identity confusion and comparisons. This is illustrated in the words of a 37-year-old Indo-European Canadian:

> I think I was about sixteen and a half or seventeen in grade twelve. We had these three day work things, where you sort of apprentice. I was interested in journalism, so I went to a radio station and you spend three days there learning about it. So, this wire came out and it mentioned the word transsexuals. It was the first time I had ever heard that word, and I guess it explained it, so I figured out "I'm not the only one in the world like this." Up to that time, I thought I was the only living person on the planet.

Some people will immediately accept that they are transsexed or transgendered and run through the next four steps in a matter of seconds. They will more or less immediately, and with great relief, accept that they are transsexed or transgendered. Others may take many years to come to terms with their feelings.

STAGE 5: IDENTITY CONFUSION ABOUT TRANSSEXUALISM OR TRANSGENDERISM

Most people who will one day identify as transsexed or transgendered recall their discovery of transsexualism or transgenderism as a significant event in their lives. Such people may not immediately begin to actively engage with the idea as an option for themselves. They may retain the idea as a precious touchstone to which they return from time to time until they are prepared to begin to consider its relevance to their own lives. Over time, the idea of transsexualism or transgenderism takes on more and more significance and they begin to wonder if they might be transsexed or transgendered themselves, thus entering a stage of identity confusion.

In order to help with the identity confusion that such questions engender, people will begin to seek out further information about exactly what it might mean to be transsexed or transgendered. Thus they will begin to engage in a deeper level of both external and internal inquiry as a response to their initial discoveries.

For further information, most people will turn to the Internet, where they will find a plethora of resources available to them: everything from reading lists and on-line bookstores to chat rooms to graphic photos and descriptions of medical procedures. When the information garnered seems that it might apply, individuals may begin to more seriously entertain the idea that they might be transsexed or transgendered. The opening of this possibility leads to the next stage: identity comparisons.

STAGE 6: IDENTITY COMPARISONS
ABOUT TRANSSEXUALISM OR TRANSGENDERISM

Once individuals have begun to entertain the possibility that they might be transsexed or transgendered, the next step is to try to come to a more definitive conclusion. At this stage the focus is on comparisons between oneself and transsexed and transgendered people, between oneself and people from one's originally assigned gender and sex, and between oneself and people of the gender and sex to which one might be moving. The point of these comparisons is to determine which comparisons provide better likenesses.

During this stage, people who will one day identify as female-to-male transsexed or transgendered will increasingly find that they have more in common with men and female-to-male transsexed and transgendered people than with women. By the time persons reach this stage it is highly likely that they have already largely abandoned any attempt to identify with feminine women. Thus their starting point will most likely be in their identities as masculine women, often as butch lesbians. When they make such comparisons they increasingly focus their attention on the ways that they feel alienated and different from those who once were their reference group. Increasingly they find that the concerns of women do not mirror their own whereas those of men increasingly do. When they weigh the results of these comparisons against what they know of female-to-male transsexed and transgendered people, they find that those comparisons progressively reveal more and more congruencies. As they start to recognize that they may be transsexed or transgendered, they will simultaneously start to disengage from their identities as women and as females. This process is illustrated in the words of a 34-year-old white telemarketer who said:

> I latched on to the lesbian community. So I had to de-emphasize certain aspects of myself. I felt that I was male but, because I had decided that the lesbian community was the only place that I could ever begin to fit in in a sexual context, I really felt that I was being dishonest because I was pretending to be female identified, but I really wasn't. And they usually picked up on it. Ever since I discovered lesbianism, the standard line has been "But you're different. You're not a dyke. You don't seem like a lesbian."

Male-to-female persons tend to go through very similar processes at this stage. There are, however, some important differences. Those who will come to identify as transsexed or transgendered may come to their identity comparisons about transsexualism or transgenderism from two somewhat different directions. In one way, many male-to-female people are similar to their female-to-male counterparts in that, by the time they reach this stage, they will have been living as feminine men for some time. They will have largely given up attempting to perform stereotypical masculinity and will have been living as openly very feminine men. When they make comparisons between themselves and women, and between themselves and transsexed and transgendered people, they find themselves better reflected than when they compare themselves to stereotypical men.

Another group of males who come to this stage come to it through a different route. A sizable minority of males come to this stage after many years of living a unremarkably masculine public life while maintaining a private feminine persona complete with name, clothing, make-up, hairstyles, accessories, and possibly a social circle as well. Those males who privately crossdress and who have had some contact with others of similar predilections are likely to have felt mirrored by them and to have already adopted a transgendered identity. Thus their identity comparisons are between their own experiences "*en femme*" and those of women, and male-to-female transsexed and transgendered people. Some may feel satisfied with transgendered as an apt description of who they are. Others may feel that to be insufficient and may move into the next stage of exploration.

STAGE 7: TOLERANCE
OF TRANSSEXUAL OR TRANSGENDERED IDENTITY

For some people, the stages of identity comparison and identity tolerance are very brief and overlapping. For them, the relief offered by the possibility of a transsexual or transgendered identity is so great that they are able to come to a rapid tolerance or even acceptance of that identity almost as soon as they become aware of it. For most people, however, taking on such an identity is a more gradual process. After learning of transsexualism or transgenderism and going through stages of confusion and comparison, most individuals who come to identify themselves as transsexed or transgendered will come to a stage of identity tolerance wherein they begin to accept that the label of transsexual or transgendered probably is a fitting description of who they are. This in-between stage of "I am probably transsexual" or "I am probably transgendered" is used by many people as an avenue to allow them to come to terms with the enormity of what it means to identify oneself as transsexed or transgendered. During this and the next stage, people more thoroughly disengage from the gender and sex to which they were assigned at birth. Those who are coming to identify as transsexed start to be able to say to themselves and to others that they are probably headed toward a change of gender and of sex. It is during this stage that the identity of transsexual or transgendered starts to take prominence over any other. One 49-year-old white transgendered musician spoke of the process this way:

I already felt I was weird enough. This sounds cruel. I don't mean it to, but you gotta admit there's something sideshow freakish about it. You know, all these men–big guys with beards wearing lipstick and the long hair . . . I saw a lot of sadness and damage and things I'd never seen before, and I felt like: "Am I just going to be a freak all my life, and live in this underworld of freakishness all the time? They're nice people, but is this going to be my whole life? Am I just going to lose all my friends and all the other life I had that I treasured and valued, and just forever be some kind of a weirdo?"

That was just an initial thing. I got to know these people, and I saw them as real human beings, and I knew that I just didn't want to be that way myself, and I felt like that was going to be the rest of my life, and it was a very dismal, bleak outlook for me. 'Cause I saw how damaged they were, and how inconclusive everything was, how long it took, and maybe a lot of times people wouldn't make it. And even if they did, it would never be complete. I saw all the negative sides of it first, and then after that, I got more and more self-determination or something, more in control of my mind and my outlook and felt more at home with it, and began to balance out again. I went through a lot of different funny, bumpy stages with it.

STAGE 8: DELAY BEFORE ACCEPTANCE OF TRANSSEXUAL OR TRANSGENDERED IDENTITY

Many people who are on their way to accepting themselves as transsexed or transgendered enter into a period of delay until they have enough information about themselves and about transsexualism or transgenderism that they can be sure that it offers them the correct solution to their gender discomfort. During this stage of delay, individuals engage in various techniques of reality testing to see if they can fully embrace an identity which until this time they were merely tolerating as a possibility (Diamond, 1997).

Individuals searching for an identity which can bring them to peace within themselves need to feel that they are seen for who they are. At this stage, they especially need others who are sufficiently different from themselves that they can act as impartial expert witnesses who can validate that what they feel like on the inside is real enough to be perceptible by others. They also particularly need others who are similar enough to themselves that they can mirror back to them a confirmatory likeness which says, "You are one of us."

Intimate emotional and/or sexual relationships is one major arena of such reality testing. When loved ones and/or sexual partners are able to witness the validity of both the rejection of the old identity and the adoption of the new identity, individuals are more able to move into a full-scale adoption of a transsexed or transgendered identity. Female-bodied individuals who are doing this kind of reality testing often find valued witnessing of their incipient transsexual or transgendered identities when their sexual/romantic partners have a history of attractions to men or otherwise find the questioning individual to be more like a man than not. Male-bodied people may follow a similar kind of exploration but are less commonly able to receive witnessing of their gender identity within already established relationships with either women or men and are more likely to have to rely on more fleeting or superficial kinds of relations such as flirtations or anonymous sexual encounters for their confirmations.

When intimates are unable to provide that kind of witnessing, people may tarry longer in the stage of delay, perhaps temporarily choosing some other descriptive label for themselves, such as queer. Conversely, when a relationship predicated on one's originally assigned sex and gender does not work out, individuals may also see the reason for the failure as being grounded in inappropriateness of their originally assigned sex and gender. They may then take their inability to make the relationship work as a confirmation of their transsexualism or transgenderism, jettison the relationship, and move more determinedly into a transsexed or transgendered identity. In the words of a 31-year-old white transman construction worker:

> Being with women, the feedback I got, the love I got was towards the physical woman. And for me, that was a conflict sexually, 'cause I felt different sexually. Making love from my heart, I was not making love as a woman with a woman. From my heart, it was that I was a male. It's a completely different dynamic. Also it depends on whether you make love with a lesbian or a heterosexual woman. Most of my lovers in my relationships were heterosexual women, and the difference–it's hard to explain cause it's just a different dynamic entirely on a feeling level– there is a different approach from a woman to her man than the approach from one woman to another woman who are lovers. It comes out in power differences.

People at this stage also turn to transsexed and transgendered people for a mirroring confirmation of their transsexualism or transgenderism. Those individuals who are fortunate enough to make contact with transsexed and transgendered people through support groups, the Internet, social contacts, or conferences have an invaluable resource available to them. Through various kinds of self-revealing discussions, they can avail themselves of the opportunity to compare their own feelings and experiences with those of people who have already adopted a transsexed or transgendered identity. When they find themselves mirrored in these comparisons, they can begin to reach more definitive conclusions about their own identities. Although not everyone struggling with this kind of identity issue will personally know transsexed or transgendered people at this stage of their lives, they may find ways to gain access to audio, video, print, or electronic biographical, autobiographical, and professional depictions of the lives of transsexed and transgendered people. These kinds of sources are also effectively used by many people to help them to decide whether or not they really are transsexed or transgendered and what they want to do about themselves. For example, a 45-year-old white electrologist went through this kind of thinking process:

> I was about twelve [when I saw a story about a transsexual] in the headlines and I read it word for word and studied every picture and realized that she and I had an immense amount in common. The lights went off like a penny arcade. Obviously there was help for her so hopefully I would be able to do something about my problem at some point. So that was the first inkling I had that there was anyone like me and that there was some sort of resource that at some age in my life I could pursue.
>
> I was 18 or 19 when I started looking into what I could do for myself and I finally took books out of the library and could do some reading and that type of thing. Put me in touch more with my problem. The photographs were close-ups, very grisly and limited in what they could accomplish. So it was sort of another monstrous choice. Do I stay the strange, that I am with these feelings and try to muddle through for a while longer, or do I do something about it now?

The stage of delay has another function for many male-to-female people. Many males who crossdress also come to question whether they might be transsexed and also go through stages of identity confusion, identity comparisons, and identity tolerance. At any of these stages some males become overwhelmed with shame and fear about the social and psychological implications of their expressions of their femininity. Periodically those feelings become expressed in episodes of radical retreat from any expression of femininity during which time all clothing and accoutrements of femininity are purged from their lives. Many males who crossdress and never will become transsexed follow this pattern as do many who do ultimately become transsexed. It is not unusual for an individual to repeat this pattern of purging and re-approach several times over a lifetime.

STAGE 9: ACCEPTANCE
OF TRANSSEXUAL OR TRANSGENDERED IDENTITY

The full acceptance of oneself as transsexed or transgendered marks still another beginning. By the time people have reached this point, they have gathered enough information and have worked through enough of their emotional anxieties about the subject that they are able to say to themselves and to others, "I am transsexual" or "I am transgendered." For some people, this stage comes very quickly–almost simultaneously with the discovery of transsexualism or transgenderism. For others, the path to this point can be much more difficult and lengthy. For all, the implications of the acceptance of such an identity are enormous.

For some people, there is nothing but tremendous relief at finally knowing who one is and what one needs to do about it. For most people, however, the acceptance of such an identity is a much more mixed blessing. Generally, by the time people reach this stage they have complicated lives involving multiple commitments predicated on their being a particular gender and sex. The prospect of reconstituting those family, business, love, friendship, and casual relationships through a gender and sex change will be daunting to say the least. Whatever the implications may be for particular individuals, all who reach this stage are confronted with the task of whether to begin the process of transforming themselves, and if so, when and how to go about it.

STAGE 10: DELAY BEFORE TRANSITION

Having come to the decision to call oneself transsexual or transgendered is only a first step. Not everyone who comes to this realization will immediately, or ever, decide to take action on it. Not all transsexed or transgendered people undergo physical or social transitions. For a variety of reasons, such as health, family, or financial considerations, some people decide that their circumstances do not warrant changing their gender or sex, or that they will only take advantage of some of the possible transformative options. For those who do decide to proceed, commonly they experience another period of delay during which there are many practical steps which must still be accomplished.

Few people at this stage know exactly what is involved or how to go about it. They may have general information about how others have accomplished their transitions, but they must take some time to find out the minutiae of exactly what needs to be done in their own case and how to do it. Most people must make an enormous number of personal and practical arrangements. Family, friends, employers, co-workers, business associates and bureaucrats may need to be informed of the impending changes. Money will need to be saved. Arrangements will need to be made with various counselors and medical personnel. Psychic readiness must be achieved. Those individuals who have access to strong support systems during this stage may be able to move through this stage quickly. Those who have children or other work or family commitments may feel obliged to delay for years. This is illustrated in the following quote from a 44-year-old unemployed white tradesperson:

> I'm unemployed. And I'm getting scared. I still got a mortgage, etc., to meet. How am I going to do this? The other thing is, I'm not going to be working through the union. I'm not going to stay in that union and work and do this. 'Cause I could never handle the flack. I know it. So, I'm not even going to try. So, I mean, I just got really scared. So, I said, "No. I can't do this. Just forget it." But I never really did forget it, I guess. I started taking shots [again]. I'm unemployed again, but my mortgage is lower and life is short. I've already taken shots, so I've made the decision. There's nothing in the future for me as I am. I'm just going to grow older, and be more of a freak. You don't want to be a freak, but . . . there's no sense worrying yourself about something [surgery] you can't get done anyways, for monetary reasons, or whatever.

During this period of delay, transsexed and transgendered people will move further in the process of disidentification with their originally assigned gender and sex. This can be an especially trying time in its own way. At this point, individuals have come to accept themselves as transsexed or transgendered, yet the people around them may witness no outward differences. However, individuals at this stage will identify more strongly with members of the gender and sex into which they are moving and they will begin to actively engage in anticipatory socialization. By so doing they begin to learn new ways of being in the world and are able to picture themselves experiencing what it might be like to live their new lives. They may be able to incorporate some of these new skills into their pre-transition lives, but in many cases this will be impractical. The disjuncture between what individuals can foresee for themselves and what they can enact may be difficult to bear.

Female-to-male individuals have a distinct advantage over male-to-female individuals at this stage. Over the past 100 years, the efforts of feminists have created far more room for variability in female gender presentations than in male gender presentations. As a result, the socially tolerated range of gendered clothing and mannerisms available to females is much greater than that available to males. Many female-bodied persons are therefore able to become relatively adept at masculinity prior to formally embarking on a gender or sex change. Male-bodied persons do not have as large a social space open to them in which to practice their femininity and therefore, while still living as men, cannot do as extensive preparation in this regard. This can make the social aspects of transition more challenging for many male-to-female persons.

STAGE 11: TRANSITION

Having decided to make a transition, having learned what needs to be done, having told everyone who needs to be told in advance, having established or relinquished commitments as appropriate, having gotten the necessary resources lined up, transition may begin. This stage may encompass changes in social presentation of self, psychotherapy, hormonal treatments, and a variety of surgeries which together accomplish gender and sex reassignment. Some people will feel that they have begun transition as soon as they make the mental decision to do so. Others will feel that transition begins only when they start psychotherapy or when they start to make observable changes to their presentation.

Different individuals engage in different strategies for transition. Some will opt for the minimum that will effect a change in how they are perceived by others. Others will require every kind of transformation possible before they will feel completely transitioned. Some people will feel that they have completed transition as soon as they find themselves consistently witnessed and mirrored as the gender and sex with which they identify. Others will feel that they are still in transition until they have completed all desired hormonal and surgical transformations. This can mean that the transition stage can be very short for those who can make a satisfactory transition entirely through changes to their social presentation, or it can last many years for individuals who require complete hormonal and surgical transitions.

Transition can be both an exhilarating and a trying stage. During this stage, individuals can spend long stretches of time during which their gender and sex are not easily recognizable to themselves or to others. On the one hand, to not know who one is, to not be known as who one is, can be extremely unsettling and difficult. On the other hand, to daily watch oneself moving out of a life which has been an enduring source of anxiety and into a life which promises to be more authentic and fulfilling can be a source of great wonder and joy.

Transition also means the leaving behind of a way of life. This departure from the total experience that comprises living as a woman or a man can be felt as a kind of death of a huge part of oneself. Thus, transition also frequently brings with it a kind of grieving for the person that one once was but no longer will be. The melancholy which accompanies this farewell can be difficult to recognize or acknowledge because individuals may feel that to do so would be to cast doubts upon the authenticity of their commitment to transitioning.

During the transition stage all kinds of normally routine activities such as shopping, eating in a restaurant, or using public lavatories can become a source of anxiety. Every interaction with persons who are unaware of or unsympathetic to an individual's transition process can be fraught with uncertainty and potential upset. Members of the general public are unaccustomed to dealing with transgendered people and may become hostile to those whom they may perceive as fraudulent or mentally ill. Although few people will react in ways which are directly dangerous to people in transition, that ever-present potential and the fact that some people do, often leaves people in transition feeling fearful, withdrawn, and defensive during parts of this stage.

However, during transition people can also become dramatically invigorated by the magnitude of the transformational changes they are undergoing. After living a lifetime being unable to fully express themselves, they feel themselves to be finally righting what has been so wrong in their lives. As other people start to see them as they see themselves, the confirmation of having their self-image witnessed and mirrored back to them can feel like a beacon in a darkness which has too often dominated their lives to that point.

During this stage the effects of testosterone are particularly salient. People transitioning from female to male benefit in their everyday lives from the relatively rapid and dramatic effects of testosterone treatments which lower their voices, increase muscle mass, and change hair growth patterns on their faces, bodies, and heads. These effects mean that female-to-male individuals are able to become socially recognized as male relatively quickly and often without the necessity of surgical procedures. This can mean that those people who take full advantage of opportunities for extensive anticipatory socialization and who respond well to testosterone treatments can have a fairly smooth and rapid social transition from everyday lives as women to everyday lives as men.

The same can less often be said of those transitioning from male to female. Most often they do so after their bodies have spent decades under the influence of testosterone, the physical effects of which are not undone by estrogen treatments. Their difficult-to-disguise masculinized secondary sex characteristics combined with less extensive opportunities for anticipatory socialization often translates into more initial difficulties in accomplishing a credible transition into unremarkable women. However, many male-to-female persons are able, with the assistance of hormonal treatments, to live quite successfully as women while awaiting other surgeries.

When it comes to surgical transitioning procedures, generally a satisfactory basic surgical transformation from male to female can be accomplished in a single surgical session, whereas the same cannot be said of female-to-male conversion. Female-to-male transformations are accomplished through a series of surgical sessions which frequently span years and rarely provide a satisfactory genital result. Furthermore, due to the scarcity of satisfactory genital surgery, many female-to-male transsexed people do not opt to undergo genital surgery. Therefore, lacking credibly male genitalia, it can be difficult for some female-to-male transsexed people to ever feel that they have satisfactorily completed their physical transitions.

STAGE 12: ACCEPTANCE
OF POST-TRANSITION GENDER/SEX IDENTITY

Transition need not be completely accomplished for a person to start to accept themselves as the gender and sex into which they are transitioning. For many people, the acceptance of a transsexed identity is identical with the acceptance of themselves as actually being a member of another gender and sex even if their bodies and lives do not yet display that truth to others. Many people, however, do require more concrete evidence before they are able to accept that they have arrived on the other side of the great gender divide. At first, their sense of themselves as their reassigned gender may seem somewhat fraudulent or artificial even to themselves. They may feel that their claim to membership is unsteady and easily challengeable due to the recentness of their transition, because of the approximate nature of their physical transitions, and because of the fact that they required transitional procedures to gain them their claim in the first place.

Over a period of months and years, individuals living as their new gender and sex learn to more deeply and profoundly understand what it means to be a person of that gender. As they accumulate a greater storehouse of experiences their sense of themselves as truly and authentically a member of their reassigned gender becomes deeper and more stable. Furthermore, as time passes and they find that they are readily and routinely witnessed and mirrored as who they feel themselves to be, many of the old anxieties and fears finally slip away to be replaced by a more serene self-acceptance than had ever before been possible. Many people find that their feelings of gender *dysphoria* are supplanted by feelings of gender *euphoria*.

STAGE 13: INTEGRATION

Most people who have undergone gender and sex transitions become seamlessly integrated into society at large. This is usually a gradual process, although it is generally more readily accomplished by female-to-male than male-to-female individuals. As transsexed people become more able and more comfortable functioning as unremarkable men and women in their everyday lives, the facts of their transitions and of their transsexuality become less salient. As time passes and as transsexed people become more firmly embedded in their post-transition lives, they and most of the people around them will tend to allow the past to recede until it only rarely intrudes upon life in the here and now. The following story from a white 37-year-old student illustrates this process of coming to greater comfort in the new life:

I always feel male, though I'm not often certain as to what that actually means. The first feeling that comes to mind is fear, fear that I don't live up to being male, don't satisfactorily meet the requirements of the role. The second feeling that comes to mind is confusion or ambivalence. I'm not often sure as to what I'm supposed to do/feel as a male. I feel I must be competent in all areas. In other words, my maleness all too often has been represented by the workaholic, Type A personality. These days I believe I am a bit more integrated. It simply ceases to be the main focus of my life. I no longer have to prove to society that I am male in order to obtain a validating mirror.

However no one can erase or escape their past. Our histories are always with us. Once one has become transsexed, once one has undergone a gender and sex transition, that is an indelible fact which will have to be managed forever. Even after full integration back into society in a transformed gender and sex status, transsexed persons will always have to pay attention to how information about their transsexuality becomes available to others. No matter how well integrated they may become, there remain many levels of disadvantages and dangers attendant upon being transsexed. Thus, for the foreseeable future, all transsexed individuals will have to face the challenge of stigma management. One 41-year-old writer described it this way:

There are times when I choose not to talk about it because there is no point. Like I'm not going to tell the gas station attendant, you know. But if it comes up, then I do talk about it freely and I'm perfectly willing to answer questions, any questions. It was a scary thing to do and it's still a scary thing, like I still don't know how the future is going to be. When I'm wondering, should I come out, I worry that people are going to stop taking me seriously, that they're going to think that I'm crazy, that they're going to think I'm disgusting, they're not going to accept me, those kinds of things. Those are really fleeting fears and so far I've been able to just press through.

Integration also takes place on another level. As the post-transition years elapse, many transsexed individuals come to better appreciate that they have found great benefits in the lessons of the first parts of their lives. Many people find that although a gender and sex transition was the right choice for them, they do not wish to abandon all of their connections to their previous lives.

At first, while identity acceptance is still becoming firmly established, any hint of one's previous way of life may seem as a threat to the establishment of a credible post-transition identity. Fears of undermining the effectiveness of one's self-presentation may prevent newly transitioning individuals from integrating aspects of their previous gender into their post-transition lives. However, it is not uncommon for those who have sufficiently consolidated their post-transition identities to re-introduce or give greater exposure to those aspects of their pre-transition lives which they still hold dear. Thus, many post-transition individuals find their way to a more comfortable type of androgyny than they could have ever entertained in their originally assigned gender and sex. In other words, once they find themselves firmly established in the right gender and sex they also find themselves able to create a life for themselves which allows them to integrate their pasts with their post-transition lives.

STAGE 14: PRIDE

Pride, as it is used here, implies both a personal sense of pride in oneself and a political stance. Persons who exhibit trans identity pride are open about their transsexualism or transgenderism in situations where it is relevant and speak up on behalf of transsexed and transgendered people when an occasion lends itself to such advocacy. Some people who demonstrate trans identity pride make working for transgender political rights the focus of their lives, whereas many others more quietly and privately work toward greater social understanding and acceptance.

Those transsexed and transgendered people who achieve a sense of pride in themselves do so against a backdrop of widespread fear, intolerance, and hostility toward transpeople. The pride of transsexed and transgendered people thus has to be seen as a ongoing accomplishment in the face of the relentless shaming that society most frequently inflicts upon transgendered people. Until such time as society at large achieves greater gender integration, the achievement and maintenance of identity pride of transpeople as a whole and as individuals will require continual effort and vigilance.

As with many of the other stages in this model, the pride stage can co-exist with ostensibly earlier stages. Individuals may feel and enact pride in their originally assigned gender and sex or in their post-transition gender and sex, they may feel pride during stages of confusion, comparison, tolerance, acceptance, delay, transition or integration. At any of these stages, transgendered people may take pride in themselves for having the courage and integrity to pursue their own very special journey. One 34-year-old white collar worker summed these feelings up nicely:

> I am proud I had the courage to do it. It's always hard to first explain it to someone because there are so many misconceptions to try to dispel. I basically feel good I had the guts to make my dream come true and to overcome the huge obstacles one overcomes when you embark on the journey of gender change. I'm proud I confronted a problem that seemed insurmountable.

CONCLUSIONS

The stages of self-discovery and self-actualization through which transsexed and transgendered people go are not unique to them alone. Many people in many walks of life go through profound transitions through which they remake themselves into someone apparently different from who they once were. Some of these transitions follow well-worn paths. Others are more exceptional and therefore more challenging to those who undergo them and to those who witness them. Those who come to know themselves as transsexed and transgendered must confront some of society's most deeply entrenched belief systems and fears in order to become themselves. In so doing they must also face their own internalizations of those values and anxieties. To come to know oneself as transsexed or transgendered requires self-examination, bravery, and naked honesty. Being/becoming transsexed or transgendered is never an easy process.

REFERENCES

Cass, V.C. (1979), Homosexual identity formation: A theoretical model. *J. Homosexuality*, 4:219-235.

_____ (1984), Homosexual identity formation: Testing a theoretical model. *J. Sex Res.*, 20:143-167.

_____ (1990), The implications of homosexual identity formation for the Kinsey model and scale of sexual preference. In: *Homosexuality/Heterosexuality: Concepts of Sexual Orientation*, eds. D.P. McWhirter, S.A. Sanders & J.M. Reinisch. New York: Oxford University Press, pp. 239-266.

Devor, H. (1987), Gender blending females: Women and sometimes men. *Amer. Behavioral Scientist*, 31:12-40.

_____ (1989), *Gender Blending: Confronting the Limits of Duality*. Bloomington, IN: Indiana University Press.

_____ (1993), Sexual orientations, identities, attractions, and practices of female-to-male transsexuals. *J. Sex Res.*, 30:303-315.

_____ (1994), Transsexualism, dissociation, and child abuse: An initial discussion based on nonclinical data. *J. Psychology & Human Sexuality*, 6:49-72.

_____ (1997a), *FTM: Female-to-Male Transsexuals in Society*. Bloomington, IN: Indiana University Press.

_____ (1997b), More than manly women: How female-to-male transsexuals reject lesbian identities. In: *Gender Blending,* eds. B. Bullough, V. Bullough & J. Elias. Amherst, NY: Prometheus, pp. 87-102.

_____ (1997c), Female gender dysphoria: Personal problem or social problem? *The Annual Review of Sex Research*, 7:44-89. Mount Vernon, IA: The Society for the Scientific Study of Sexuality.

Diamond, M. (1997), Sexual identity and sexual orientation in children with traumatized or ambiguous genitalia. *J Sex Res.*, 34:199-211.

Ebaugh, H.R.F. (1988), *Becoming an Ex: The Process of Role Exit.* Chicago: University of Chicago Press.

Fausto-Sterling, A. (2000), *Sexing the Body: Gender, Politics, and the Construction of Sexuality.* New York: Basic Books.

Kendal, M., Devor, H. & Strapko, N. (1997), Feminist and lesbian opinions about transsexuals. In: *Gender Blending,* eds. B. Bullough, V. Bullough & J. Elias. Amherst, NY: Prometheus, pp. 146-159.

Kohut, H. (1984), *How Does Analysis Cure?* Chicago: University of Chicago Press.

Laqueur, T. (1990), *Making Sex: Body and Gender from the Greeks to Freud.* Cambridge, MA: Harvard University Press.

Meyer, W. III (Chairperson), Bockting, W., Cohen-Kettenis, P., Coleman, E., DiCeglie, D., Devor, H., Gooren, L., Hage, J, Kirk, S., Kuiper, B., Laub, D., Lawrence, A., Menard, Y., Patton, J., Schaefer, L., Webb, A. & Wheeler, C. (2001), The standards of care for gender identity disorders–Sixth version. *Internat. J. Transgenderism 5:* Online at *http://www.symposion.com/ijt/soc_2001/index.htm.*

Poland, W.S. (2000), The analyst's witnessing and otherness. *J. Amer. Psychoanal. Assn.*, 48:80-93.

Tully, B. (1992), *Accounting for Transsexualism & Transhomosexuality: The Gender Identity Careers of Over 200 Men and Women.* London: Whiting & Birch.

Zucker, K.J. & Bradley, S.J. (1995), *Gender Identity Disorder and Psychosexual Problems in Children.* New York: Guilford Press.

Autogynephilia:
A Paraphilic Model
of Gender Identity Disorder

Anne A. Lawrence, MD, PhD

SUMMARY. Autogynephilia is defined as a male's propensity to be sexually aroused by the thought or image of himself as female. Autogynephilia explains the desire for sex reassignment of some male-to-female (MTF) transsexuals. It can be conceptualized as both a paraphilia and a sexual orientation. The concept of autogynephilia provides an alternative to the traditional model of transsexualism that emphasizes gender identity. Autogynephilia helps explain mid-life MTF gender transition, progression from transvestism to transsexualism, the prevalence of other paraphilias among MTF transsexuals, and late development of sexual interest in male partners. Hormone therapy and sex reassignment surgery can be effective treatments in autogynephilic transsexualism. The concept of autogynephilia can help clinicians better understand MTF transsexual clients who recognize a strong sexual component to their gender dysphoria. *[Article copies available for a fee from The Haworth Document Delivery Service: 1-800-HAWORTH. E-mail address: <docdelivery@haworthpress.com> Website: <http://www.HaworthPress.com> © 2004 by The Haworth Press, Inc. All rights reserved.]*

Anne A. Lawrence is an Associate Member of the International Academy of Sex Research, and serves on the Board of Directors of the Society for the Scientific Study of Sexuality. She has a private practice in clinical sexology in Seattle, WA.

Address correspondence to: Anne A. Lawrence, MD, PhD, 1812 E. Madison Street, Suite 102, Seattle, WA 98122-2876 (E-mail: alawrence@mindspring.com).

[Haworth co-indexing entry note]: "Autogynephilia: A Paraphilic Model of Gender Identity Disorder." Lawrence, Anne A. Co-published simultaneously in *Journal of Gay & Lesbian Psychotherapy* (The Haworth Medical Press, an imprint of The Haworth Press, Inc.) Vol. 8, No. 1/2, 2004, pp. 69-87; and: *Transgender Subjectivities: A Clinician's Guide* (ed: Ubaldo Leli, and Jack Drescher) The Haworth Medical Press, an imprint of The Haworth Press, Inc., 2004, pp. 69-87. Single or multiple copies of this article are available for a fee from The Haworth Document Delivery Service [1-800-HAWORTH, 9:00 a.m. - 5:00 p.m. (EST). E-mail address: docdelivery@haworthpress.com].

KEYWORDS. Arousal, autogynephilia, cross-dressing, gender dysphoria, gender identity, paraphilia, sex reassignment, sexual orientation, transsexual, transvestism

Biologic males who seek sex reassignment–male-to-female (MTF) transsexuals–are a diverse group. Some males who seek sex reassignment seem to fit the "classic" transsexual pattern. They were extremely feminine as children, are extremely feminine as adults, and are unambiguously attracted to men. Typically these individuals pass very easily as women, and their motivations for seeking sex reassignment seem obvious.

But other MTF transsexuals do not conform to the classic pattern. Often these individuals seek sex reassignment in their 30s, 40s, 50s, or even later, after having lived outwardly successful lives as men. Usually they were not especially feminine as children, and many are not especially feminine as adults, either. Often they have been married to females and have fathered children. Many identify as lesbian or bisexual after reassignment. Nearly all have a past or current history of sexual arousal in association with cross-dressing or cross-gender fantasy. Yet they experience gender dysphoria–a term that denotes dissatisfaction with the sexed body–as intensely as their more outwardly feminine counterparts.

Once considered rare, MTF transsexuals who do not conform to the classic pattern now appear to constitute a majority of those who seek sex reassignment (Blanchard and Sheridan, 1992), and in some large series comprise 75% or more of those who actually undergo sex reassignment surgery (SRS) (Lawrence, 2003; Muirhead-Allwood, Royle, and Young, 1999). What motivates these individuals? Why would males who have been fairly successful as men, who are not especially feminine, and who are attracted to women seek sex reassignment?

One controversial model proposes that these transsexuals suffer from a paraphilia, and that their desire for sex reassignment is the outgrowth of their paraphilic wish to look like and behave as females. This paraphilia is called *autogynephilia*. The newest revision of the *Diagnostic and Statistical Manual of Mental Disorders* (*DSM-IV-TR*) (American Psychiatric Association [APA], 2000) briefly mentions autogynephilia (p. 578), but the concept is not widely understood or appreciated, even among clinicians who routinely work with gender patients. This paper will provide an introduction to the concept of autogynephilia and will discuss its value for understanding the phenomenology, prognosis, and treatment of gender identity disorders and related conditions.

BLANCHARD'S CONCEPT OF AUTOGYNEPHILIA

The term *autogynephilia* (literally, "love of oneself as a woman") was coined in 1989 by Ray Blanchard, a clinical psychologist at the Clarke Institute of Psychiatry in Toronto (Blanchard, 1989a). Blanchard formally defined autogynephilia as "a male's propensity to be sexually aroused by the thought or image of himself as a female" (Blanchard, 1991). In a remarkable series of papers (Blanchard, 1985, 1987, 1988, 1989a, 1989b, 1991, 1992, 1993a, 1993b, 1993c; Blanchard and Clemmensen, 1988; Blanchard, Clemmensen, and Steiner, 1985, 1987), he explored the role of autogynephilia in the erotic lives of hundreds of male gender dysphoric patients.

Like many previous researchers, Blanchard was interested in the nosology of male-to-female transsexualism. Clinicians had long been aware that males who sought sex reassignment were not a homogeneous group. Several different categories of male-to-female transsexualism had been proposed, typically based on sexual orientation, history of sexual arousal to cross-dressing, or a combination of these (for reviews see Blanchard, 1989a, and Lawrence, 2003). Many observers had noted that gender dysphoric males nearly always displayed one of two uncommon erotic preferences: either exclusive sexual attraction to males, or a history of sexual arousal to cross-dressing or cross-gender fantasy (Freund, Steiner, and Chan, 1982).

Based on his research, Blanchard (1989b) concluded that there were two distinct categories of gender dysphoric males: an *androphilic* group, those who were sexually aroused exclusively or almost exclusively by males; and a nonandrophilic group, who were, or had once been, sexually aroused primarily by the idea of being female. Blanchard called this latter group *autogynephilic*: having the propensity to be sexually aroused by the thought or image of oneself as female.

His research revealed that gender dysphoric males who were primarily attracted to men (androphilic) usually reported having been quite feminine as children (Blanchard, 1988). They first presented clinically at an average age of 26 years (Blanchard, Clemmensen, and Steiner, 1987). Only about 15% of them gave any history of sexual arousal with cross-dressing (Blanchard, 1985), and generally they did not tend to be sexually aroused by fantasies of simply being female (Blanchard, 1989b).

Blanchard's other category of gender dysphoric males included those attracted primarily to women (*gynephilic*); those attracted to both women and men (bisexual); and those with little attraction to other persons of either sex (*analloerotic*, "not attracted to other people"). Blanchard (1988) found that the males in this combined group reported less childhood femininity than those in the androphilic group; some might not have been especially masculine as children, but few if any had been extremely feminine. Those in the combined group presented for initial evaluation later in life, at an average age of 34 years (Blanchard, Clemmensen, and Steiner, 1987). About 75% of them admitted to a history of sexual arousal with cross-dressing (Blanchard, 1985). Most significantly for Blanchard's theory, they were far more likely than persons in the androphilic group to be sexually aroused by autogynephilic fantasies, that is, by fantasies of simply being female (Blanchard, 1989b).

There is good reason to believe that the males in the combined group might have underreported their sexual arousal to cross-dressing. Blanchard, Clemmensen, and Steiner (1985) demonstrated that in nonandrophilic gender dysphoric males, denial of sexual arousal to cross-dressing was significantly correlated with the tendency to describe oneself in a socially approved way, as measured by the Crowne-Marlowe Social Desirability Scale. Androphilic gender dysphoric males did not show such a correlation. Moreover, Blanchard, Racansky, and Steiner (1986) demonstrated using penile plethysmography that many nonandrophilic male gender patients who denied sexual arousal to cross-dressing actually did become aroused while listening to spoken descriptions of cross-dressing scenarios. Therefore, it seems reasonable to assume that in Blanchard's combined group, a history of autogynephilic sexual arousal was nearly universal.

> Autogynephilia denotes the *propensity* to be sexually aroused by the thought or image of oneself as female. The actual occurrence and extent of such arousal will vary with time and circumstance. In autogynephilic persons, the relationship between the cross-gender stimulus and sexual excitement is probabilistic rather than inevitable. An autogynephile does not necessarily become sexually aroused every time he pictures himself as a female or engages in feminine behavior, any more than a heterosexual man automatically gets an erection whenever he sees an attractive woman. Thus, the concept of autogynephilia–like that of heterosexuality, homosexuality, or pedophilia–refers to a *potential* for sexual excitation. (Blanchard, 1991)

ANATOMIC AUTOGYNEPHILIA AND THE DESIRE FOR SRS

Blanchard (1991) formally distinguished four different types of autogynephilia in gender dysphoric males, although most of his patients demonstrated more than one type. The first type was *transvestic* autogynephilia, which denotes arousal to the act or fantasy of wearing women's clothing. Persons in whom this type of autogynephilia predominates are referred to as cross-dressers, transvestites, or "persons with transvestic fetishism" (in *DSM-IV-TR*). The second type was *behavioral* autogynephilia, which denotes arousal to the act or fantasy of engaging in some behavior regarded as typically feminine. This behavior could range from knitting in the company of other women to having sexual intercourse with a male. The latter behavior, according to Blanchard's formulation, did not represent genuine androphilia, because the arousal was not to the male partner per se, but rather to engaging in a behavior regarded as typical of females. The third type was *physiologic* autogynephilia, which denotes arousal to fantasies such as being pregnant, menstruating, or breast-feeding. The fourth type was *anatomic* autogynephilia, which denotes arousal to the fantasy of having a woman's body, or aspects of one, such as breasts or a vulva. The relative prevalence of the different types of autogynephilia is not known, but transvestic autogynephilia appears to be the most common type. Blanchard (1991) found that 90% of transsexuals who experienced anatomic autogynephilia had also experienced transvestic autogynephilia.

It was entirely predictable, Blanchard felt, that males who experienced sexual arousal from the idea of having a woman's body would in fact seek to acquire or inhabit such a body. His research subsequently confirmed that patients with the anatomic type of autogynephilia were the ones most interested in physical transformation, including SRS (Blanchard, 1993b). He summarized his theory this way:

> Autogynephilia takes a variety of forms. Some men are most aroused sexually by the idea of wearing women's clothes, and they are primarily interested in wearing women's clothes. Some men are most aroused sexually by the idea of having a woman's body, and they are most interested in acquiring a woman's body. Viewed in this light, the desire for sex reassignment surgery of the latter group appears as logical as the desire of heterosexual men to marry wives, the desire of homosexual men to establish permanent relationships with male partners, and perhaps the desire of other paraphilic men to bond with their paraphilic objects in ways no one has thought to observe. (Blanchard, 1991)

The concept of autogynephilia provides a *model* for understanding why some individuals with a history of cross-gender eroticism might seek sex reassignment. Blanchard proposed that transsexuals with a history of autogynephilic eroticism *behave as though* they were motivated by the desire to actualize their paraphilic fantasy of feminizing their bodies. This hypothesized motivation might or might not correspond to the motivations transsexuals themselves might declare for their decisions to seek sex reassignment.

PREVALENCE OF AUTOGYNEPHILIA IN TRANSSEXUALS

It is difficult to estimate the prevalence of autogynephilic eroticism in MTF transsexuals and other transgendered persons. Data from clinical populations provide limited evidence concerning (a) the percentage of persons reporting *any* history of autogynephilic arousal, and (b) the percentage of persons reporting *current* autogynephilic arousal.

Among transsexuals who have not undergone SRS, the percentage of individuals who give any history of sexual arousal to cross-dressing or cross-gender fantasy varies considerably from study to study. Hoenig and Kenna (1974) reported one of the highest figures, 83%, while Buhrich and McConaghy (1978) reported one of the lowest, 17%. Two of the largest studies, by Blanchard (1985; $N = 163$) and by Doorn, Poortinga, and Verschoor (1994; $N = 155$), reported prevalence figures of 37% and 31%, respectively. Lawrence (2003) surveyed 232 MTF transsexuals who had undergone SRS with surgeon Toby Meltzer between 1994 and 2001; 86% of those giving a numerical response reported having experienced autogynephilic arousal at least occasionally before SRS, and 49% reported having experienced "hundreds of episodes or more" before SRS. Following SRS, over a mean duration of 3 years, 44% of those giving a numerical response reported having experienced at least a few episodes of autogynephilic arousal, but only 3% reported having experienced hundreds of episodes or more (Lawrence, unpublished paper).

Blanchard and Clemmensen (1988) studied current sexual arousal to cross-dressing in 113 males who were heterosexual relative to biologic sex and who exhibited intense gender dysphoria. All stated that they had felt like a woman at all times for at least one year, and over 97% acknowledged a desire for SRS. Over half (52%) reported that they had experienced sexual arousal with cross-dressing at least occasionally during the past year, and 15% had experienced such arousal usually or always. Nearly half (46%) reported that they had masturbated while cross-dressing at least occasionally during the past year, and 15% reported that they had masturbated on half or more of the occasions when they cross-dressed. Doorn, Poortinga, and Verschoor (1994) noted that in their group of 155 transsexual patients, 16% reported that cross-dressing was currently sexually arousing, at least at times; all of their patients were taking hormones and were seeking SRS.

There is evidence that transgendered persons tend to underreport their sexual arousal to cross-dressing and cross-gender fantasy (Blanchard, Racansky, and Steiner, 1986). Therefore, the percentages given above should probably be regarded as low-end estimates.

AUTOGYNEPHILIA AS A PARAPHILIA AND A SEXUAL ORIENTATION

Blanchard (1993c) considered autogynephilia to be a paraphilia, or unusual sexual arousal pattern. Paraphilias, as described in the *DSM-IV-TR*, are characterized by "recurrent, intense sexual urges, fantasies, or behaviors that involve unusual objects, activities, or situations and cause clinically significant distress or impairment in . . . functioning" (APA, 2000, p. 535). Blanchard was not the first clinician to propose that transsexualism might sometimes be a paraphilic phenomenon; Buhrich and McConaghy (1977), Christie Brown (1983), Freund, Steiner, and Chan (1982), Meyer (1982), and Wilson and Gosselin (1980) had previously made similar suggestions.

However, Blanchard proposed that autogynephilia could also be considered a sexual orientation:

> Autogynephilia might be better characterized as an orientation than as a paraphilia. The term *orientation* encompasses behavior, correlated with sexual behavior but distinct from it, that may ultimately have a greater impact on the life of the individual. For homosexual and heterosexual men, such correlated behavior includes courtship, love, and cohabitation with a partner of the preferred sex; for autogynephilic men, it includes the desire to achieve, with clothing, hormones, or surgery, an appearance like the preferred self-image of their erotic fantasies. (Blanchard, 1993c)

Implicit in the concept that autogynephilia is a sexual orientation as well as a paraphilia is the idea that autogynephilia encompasses more than just "autogyneroticism." The Greek word *philos* means "loving," and the term *autogynephilia* accurately implies that persons who experience it are usually genuinely *in love with* the idea of being women. To many autogynephiles, the idea of being a woman is more than just sexual arousing: it is also comforting, aesthetically pleasing, inspiring, and spiritually transformative, just as other kinds of love frequently are.

AUTOGYNEPHILIA AND GENDER DYSPHORIA

Although some transsexuals find the idea of becoming a woman sexually exciting, it would be a mistake to imagine that they are always happy about their autogynephilic feelings, or that they seek sex reassignment primarily as a hedonistic indulgence. Persons who experience severe anatomic autogynephilia often suffer greatly due to their feelings (Lawrence, 1999c). Unusual and intense sexual urges that cannot be satisfied are not pleasant (Levine, Risen, and Althof, 1990), and transsexuals frequently find their autogynephilic feelings to be unwanted, intrusive, painful, and disabling. In short, anatomic autogynephilia is often associated with severe gender dysphoria. For autogynephilic transsexuals, gender dysphoria and autogynephilic sexual desire act like different sides of the same coin (Blanchard, 1993c). Gender dysphoria provides the "push" toward sex reassignment, while autogynephilic sexual desire provides the "pull."

AUTOGYNEPHILIA, GENDER IDENTITY,
AND THE TRANSSEXUAL MOTIVE

Although Blanchard's theory provides an explanation of the desire for sex reassignment in males with a history of autogynephilic arousal, it does not purport to provide a complete or exclusive explanation. Blanchard (1991) acknowledged this explicitly:

> Gender dysphoria, in young nonhomosexual males, usually appears along with, or subsequent to, autogynephilia; in later years, however, autogynephilic sexual arousal may diminish or disappear, while the transsexual wish remains or grows even stronger. Such histories are often produced by gender dysphoric patients, but one does not have to rely on self-report to accept that *the transsexual motive may attain, or inherently possess, some independence from autogynephilia.* (emphasis added)

The traditional explanation of the transsexual motive in persons with a history of autogynephilic arousal–and in transsexuals generally–is that these individuals experience their biologic sex as incongruent with their gender identity. *Gender identity* is a term that refers to one's inner sense of being male or female, masculine or feminine. Although Blanchard's autogynephilia theory offers a different emphasis, it is not inconsistent with the traditional gender-identity-based formulation. For example, a person might experience autogynephilic eroticism and also experience discomfort with the male gender role; both factors might contribute to the person's gender dysphoria. Moreover, autogynephilic eroticism, especially if persistently and intensely experienced, could in itself contribute to the development of a cross-gender identity. According to Levine, Risen, and Althof (1990), "It is not yet widely recognized that what we want to do with our bodies . . . during sexual arousal contributes to our sexual identities. [Both paraphilic and nonparaphilic individuals] develop self-concepts from their erotic intentions." Blanchard's autogynephilia model and the traditional gender-identity-based model of transsexualism can thus be seen as complementary rather than mutually exclusive.

Several researchers and clinicians have concluded that nearly all MTF transsexuals (and many transvestites) with a history of autogynephilic arousal experience genuine cross-gender wishes, which may precede, or exist independently of, autogynephilic eroticism. Buhrich and McConaghy (1977) documented consistent self-reports of childhood gender nonconformity in 12 MTF transsexuals with a history of sexual arousal to cross-dressing. Langevin (1985) concluded that "gender identity may be as significant a component in transvestism as erotic needs." Johnson and Hunt (1990) hypothesized that autogynephilic transsexuals experience real gender identity conflicts, just as androphilic transsexuals do, but resolve these conflicts later in life. Levine

(1993) argued that autogynephilic eroticism could be an effect rather than a cause of atypical gender identity and proposed that "cross-dressing and . . . autogynephilic fantasy are the external and internal manifestations of the same phenomenon–the conscious experience of the self as at least partially female." Doorn, Poortinga, and Verschoor (1994) found that their late-onset MTF transsexual patients, 42% of whom acknowledged a past history of sexual arousal to cross-dressing, reported a high prevalence of female-typical pre-adolescent gender behaviors. Seil (1996) suggested that transsexuals with a history of sexual arousal to cross-dressing experience cross-gender feelings at an early age, just as other transsexuals do; however, they experience their cross-gender feelings as ego-dystonic rather than ego-syntonic.

In summary, while autogynephilia provides a plausible explanation of the desire for sex reassignment in males with a history of autogynephilic arousal, the traditional model that emphasizes gender nonconformity and gender identity also has plausibility in autogynephiles. Keeping both models in mind can offer the clinician a more nuanced understanding of transsexual motivation.

FEMINIZING HORMONE THERAPY AND AUTOGYNEPHILIA

Hoenig and Kenna (1974) argued that transsexualism could not represent a paraphilia, because transsexuals' desire for sex reassignment was not elimi-nated by chemical or physical castration. When autogynephilic transsexuals take feminizing hormones, their testosterone levels usually decrease dramati-cally, and their interest in genital sexuality typically declines as well. How-ever, their desire for sex reassignment usually remains unchanged.

While these observations might seem to pose a problem for Blanchard's theory, for several reasons they do not. First, very low testosterone levels do not necessarily eliminate all capacity for sexual arousal, as studies in hypo-gonadal males have shown (e.g., Kwan et al., 1983). Second, as noted earlier, some aspects of the paraphilic wish for feminization that autogynephilic trans-sexuals experience may not be contingent upon genital arousal. For example, the physical feminization produced by hormone therapy may be comforting and aesthetically pleasing to autogynephilic transsexuals, even if it is not strongly genitally arousing. Finally, reduction in the intensity of paraphilic sexual arousal might actually be welcomed by many transsexuals. As dis-cussed earlier, paraphilic arousal can sometimes be unwanted, intrusive, and ego-dystonic; reduced sexual arousal might sometimes be a relief.

Sexual arousal that acts as a reminder of unwanted male anatomy can be es-pecially distressing to transsexuals. Blanchard and Clemmensen (1988) reported that half of their informants who experienced sexual arousal to cross-dressing were sometimes bothered by this arousal. Persons who were more bothered by autogynephilic arousal were also significantly more gender dysphoric than those who were not bothered. Lawrence (1999c) proposed that one of the reasons feminizing hormone therapy is so well accepted by autogynephilic transsexuals is that it reduces serum testosterone levels and thus helps control ego-dystonic paraphilic arousal, in addition to producing desired feminization. This hypothesis is consistent with the narratives provided by some autogynephilic transsexuals (Lawrence, 1999a, #5; 1999b, #40).

SATISFACTION WITH SRS IN AUTOGYNEPHILIC TRANSSEXUALS

In the 1960s and early 1970s, any history of sexual arousal to cross-dressing or cross-gender fantasy was regarded as a contraindication to SRS (e.g., Baker, 1969). The introduction of the concept of *gender dysphoria syndrome* by Laub and Fisk (1974) liberalized the indications for SRS and made SRS more easily available to persons with a history of autogynephilic arousal. However, some experts continued to believe that sexual arousal to crossdressing or cross-gender fantasy was a contraindication to SRS (Lundström, Pauly, and Wålinder, 1984; Sørensen, 1981), or that a history of such arousal significantly increased the likelihood of postoperative regret (Landén et al., 1998). Lawrence (2003) conducted a large follow-up study of SRS outcomes, using a questionnaire that asked explicitly about respondents' history of autogynephilic arousal before SRS; this study found no significant correlation between frequency of autogynephilic arousal before SRS and postoperative regret.

EXPLANATORY VALUE OF AUTOGYNEPHILIA

Blanchard's theory of autogynephilia helps to explain several otherwise puzzling observations about MTF transsexualism. First, it convincingly explains why some men who are attracted to women, who have been fairly successful as men, and who appear unremarkably masculine would wish to undergo sex reassignment. Why would men who have been successful fighter pilots, construction workers, or captains of industry–men who seem not the least bit feminine, and who appear entirely comfortable being men–want to undergo sex reassignment? Attributing this solely to some long-hidden inner femininity might seem implausible. But if these individuals found the idea of being a woman *sexually* appealing, then their motivation would be easier to understand. The phenomenon of a middle-aged man risking his career, his reputation, and his marriage for the sake of a sexual obsession is well known. By proposing that certain types of MTF transsexualism can have sexual motivations, rather than (or in addition to) gender motivations, Blanchard's auto-gynephilia theory helps to explain this phenomenon.

Second, Blanchard's theory helps to explain the relationship between transsexualism and transvestism. Transvestism is considered to be a para-philia, or unusual pattern of sexual arousal, in the *DSM-IV-TR* (APA, 2000) and has always been classified as such in the *DSM*. However, clinicians have long recognized that some men who previously considered themselves trans-vestites eventually decide to seek SRS and live full-time as women. If trans-vestism is purely an erotic phenomenon and transsexualism is purely a gender identity phenomenon, then there is no obvious explanation for this progres-sion. But if both transvestism and some forms of MTF transsexualism are manifestations of autogynephilia–an erotic condition that also influences gen-der identity–then this progression is explained convincingly.

Third, Blanchard's autogynephilia theory helps explain why transvestism and transsexualism are often associated with other unusual erotic interests. Sexual scientists have observed for decades that unusual sexual interests–sa-domasochism, bondage, autoerotic asphyxia, interest in leather and rubber, exhibitionism, voyeurism, infantilism, pedophilia–frequently do not occur in isolation, but instead tend to co-occur. Males who have one unusual sexual in-terest are far more likely to have one or more *other* unusual sexual interests than would be expected simply by chance (Abel and Osborn, 1992; Wilson and Gosselin, 1980). Furthermore, other unusual erotic interests are very com-mon among transvestites and some MTF transsexuals. Wilson and Gosselin (1980) found that 63% of their sample of transvestites and transsexuals also described fetishistic or sadomasochistic interests. Blanchard and Hucker (1991) reported that transvestism accompanied many cases of autoerotic asphyxia. Abel and Osborn (1992) documented the co-occurrence of transvestism and transsexualism with other paraphilias. If transsexualism and transvestism are purely gender-identity-based phenomena, then these associations make no sense. But if transsexualism and transvestism sometimes represent unusual sexual interests–as Blanchard's autogynephilia theory proposes–then their as-sociation with other uncommon sexual interests does make sense.

Finally, the concept of autogynephilia helps to explain the unusual sexual fantasies that some transvestites and MTF transsexuals have concerning men, and the late development of sexual interest in male partners by some MTF transsexuals. Many heterosexual transvestites and formerly heterosexual MTF transsexuals have sexual fantasies about men, but usually these are not quite like the fantasies of genuine androphiles (Blanchard, 1989b). In the transsex-ual and transvestite fantasies there is little emphasis on the specific character-istics of the imagined male partner. Often the imagined partner is faceless or quite abstract, and seems to be present primarily to validate the femininity of the person having the fantasy, rather than as a desirable partner in his own right (Blanchard, 1991). It is also fairly common for heterosexual transvestites to engage in sex with men when cross-dressed. Why don't they do this at other times? Apparently, because the attraction is not to the male partner per se, but to the way in which acting like a woman in relationship to a man is sexually gratifying. Autogynephilia also explains why some transsexuals who were never interested in having sex with men before transition develop this interest after undergoing SRS. It is not because they have miraculously changed their underlying sexual orientation and now find men's bodies arousing. Rather, it is because they can finally actualize their autogynephilic fantasy of having sex with a male.

Some transsexuals' autogynephilic interest in male partners can appear almost indistinguishable from genuine androphilia, as the following case vignette illustrates:

> A 38-year-old biologic male who had been using estrogen without medical supervision sought monitored hormone therapy under a harm-reduction model. She had been married to a female for nine years, her past sexual experiences had been exclusively with women, and she openly identified as an autogynephilic transsexual. She was especially aroused by the idea of having sex with a man as a woman. She responded well to feminizing hormone therapy, underwent facial electrolysis and cosmetic surgery, and began living full-time in female role. She became successfully employed as a woman in a job where no one knew her past history. A few months later, she became romantically involved with a male coworker. Their sexual activity was limited to light petting, because the patient had not yet undergone SRS and had not disclosed this to her partner. She expressed a strong desire for SRS, which would enable her to have sexual intercourse with men. When asked how this fit with her earlier declaration that she was an autogynephilic transsexual, she replied that it was entirely consistent. She stated that she felt no particular attraction to men's bodies, but was only interested in the way in which being with a man sexually made her feel like a desirable woman. Asked whether this meant that her male partner functioned primarily as another "fashion accessory" with which to enhance her self-image, like a pretty dress or a designer handbag, she replied that this metaphor expressed her feelings exactly.

DENIAL OF CURRENT AUTOGYNEPHILIC AROUSAL BY TRANSSEXUALS

Although most nonandrophilic transsexuals admit that they have experienced autogynephilic arousal at some time in the past, many report that they no longer experience such arousal. If autogynephilia is really akin to a sexual orientation, this might seem surprising. Heterosexual and gay males, for example, may cease to experience sexual arousal to a particular partner, but they rarely claim that they no longer experience sexual arousal to *any* potential partners within their preferred category.

There are several possible explanations of the denial of current autogynephilic arousal by transsexuals who have a past history of such arousal. As previously noted, some males with this history who deny current sexual arousal to cross-dressing nevertheless demonstrate physiologic arousal in response to spoken cross-dressing narratives (Blanchard, Racansky, and Steiner, 1986). Some MTF transsexuals might consciously experience physiologic arousal to cross-gender behavior or fantasy, but might deny or minimize this arousal in order to present themselves in a socially approved manner. Blanchard, Clemmensen, and Steiner (1985) demonstrated a correlation between denial of autogynephilic arousal and participants' scores on the Crowne-Marlowe Social Desirability Scale, a finding that gives credence to this possibility.

Alternatively, the feelings and sensations that accompany autogynephilic arousal might sometimes be too mild to be consciously perceived, or if perceived might be interpreted as something other than sexual arousal. The mild sexual arousal that accompanies the earliest stages of the sexual response cycle (Masters and Johnson, 1966, pp. 4-7) might not be noticed by some autogynephilic individuals. Nevertheless, as Docter (1988) emphasized, "the fact that an individual reports that no sexual 'turn-on' is experienced [with cross-dressing] does not necessarily mean that no components of the sexual response pattern are operative" (p. 117). Misinterpretation of feelings of sexual arousal is another possibility. Docter (1988) proposed that "another hypothesis might be that the mild sexual arousal that may accompany. . . fetishistic cross-dressing is subjectively interpreted as calming despite what may be mild physiological arousal" (p. 117).

Finally, it is possible that some transsexuals with a history of autogynephilic arousal might genuinely cease to experience any physiologic arousal to cross-gender behavior or fantasy. Feminizing hormone therapy, which lowers testosterone levels and reduces libido, might plausibly contribute to this. If autogynephilic arousal no longer occurs in these individuals, what explains their continued wish for sex reassignment? Blanchard proposed that, after a period of time, stimuli that have been experienced as sexually gratifying might come to be regarded as rewarding and desirable, even when they no longer evoke intense genital arousal. Using the analogy of heterosexual marriage, he observed that husbands often continue to experience a deep emotional connection to their wives, even after their initial intense sexual attraction has diminished or completely disappeared (Blanchard, 1991). This is consistent with the point made earlier: autogynephilic persons can be seen as being in love with the idea of being women, and this love might plausibly persist even after physiologic arousal disappears.

CONTROVERSY AMONG TRANSSEXUALS CONCERNING AUTOGYNEPHILIA

Clinicians should be aware that the concept of autogynephilia is controversial among MTF transsexuals. Some find the concept to be consistent with their identities, validating, and liberating. Others find it to be inconsistent with their identities, pejorative, and stigmatizing.

Blanchard's autogynephilia model was designed to help explain transgendered persons' behavior, such as their patterns of sexual arousal and activity, their partner choices, and their requests for medical and surgical interventions. It was not designed to explain transgendered persons' identities or their stated motivations for seeking SRS. However, as MTF transsexuals have become aware of Blanchard's model from articles in popular magazines such as *Transgender Tapestry* (Lawrence, 1998, 2000), they have begun to express their opinions about autogynephilia and the extent to which the model based on it is or is not consistent with their feelings and identities.

Some MTF transsexuals and other transgendered persons who appear to conform to the autogynephilic profile clearly state that the autogynephilia model is *not* consistent with their personal experiences and identities (e.g., Allison, 2001; Barnes, 2001; Buckwalter, 2001). These individuals typically report that they no longer experience autogynephilic arousal (or occasionally that they never did), or that autogynephilia did not play a significant part in their decisions to undergo gender transition and SRS. For example, Allison (2001) states:

> We have sacrificed so much for the validation of our personal identity. We didn't do it for sexual desire . . . We did it to relieve our own discomfort and live the rest of our lives in the role that is right for us.

Other transsexuals tell a different story. They report that Blanchard's autogynephilia model accurately describes their experiences and motivations, and that they are grateful to learn that there is a theory that speaks to their experience. Lawrence (1999a, 1999b) has collected dozens of such narratives. One anonymous transsexual informant writes as follows:

> I have yet to read an explanation . . . that more closely and accurately describes the motivation I feel than . . . autogynephilia. I have known since very early childhood that I was transsexual . . . However, the standard or classic transsexual definitions did not seem to apply. This is the first time

anybody has ever said it is OK to have sexual feelings and motives . . . I have been reluctant to proceed, [but] now with what I have learned, I will approach counseling with a new zeal. Thank you so much for bringing this much needed information to light. (Lawrence, 1999b, #34)

As the concept of autogynephilia becomes better known among transsexuals, it is likely that more patients will discuss the issue with professionals. Clinicians may be called upon to dispel misconceptions about Blanchard's autogynephilia model. It may be helpful to reassure patients that (a) the autogynephilia model attempts to explain behavior, but does not attempt to explain individuals' identities; (b) the model does not imply that transsexualism is exclusively about sex; and (c) autogynephilia is not the basis for deciding whether someone is, or is not, a "real" transsexual.

UNRESOLVED QUESTIONS CONCERNING AUTOGYNEPHILIA

It remains unclear whether autogynephilia genuinely occurs in androphilic transsexuals, and if so, what implications this might have for Blanchard's model. Some studies have reported prevalence rates of autogynephilia ranging from 10% to 36% among androphilic gender dysphoric males (Bentler, 1976; Blanchard, 1985; Blanchard, Clemmensen, and Steiner, 1987; Freund, Steiner, and Chan, 1982; Leavitt and Berger, 1990). Blanchard (1985) proposed that some supposedly androphilic individuals who admitted to autogynephilic arousal were probably not genuinely androphilic, but had misrepresented their sexual orientation in order to appear more classically transsexual. However, it is not clear why such individuals would then admit to autogynephilic arousal, which is surely not a classically transsexual trait.

Some transsexuals who freely acknowledge a history of autogynephilia report that they experienced cross-gender wishes long before they experienced autogynephilic arousal. It is unclear whether such reports are accurate, and if so, what their implications might be for Blanchard's theory. Typically, these individuals report that their cross-gender wishes began in early childhood, but that they did not experience autogynephilic arousal until puberty. It is possible that these individuals might actually have experienced autogynephilic arousal earlier, but either did not remember it, or did not interpret it as sexual arousal. Case reports by Stoller (1985) and by Zucker and Blanchard (1997) make it clear that genital arousal with cross-dressing can occur as early as age 3 years. Nevertheless, it remains possible that cross-gender wishes might sometimes precede autogynephilic arousal by many years. This suggests the possibility that autogynephilia might sometimes be an effect rather than a cause of gender dysphoria. Since there is no accepted theory that explains how *any* erotic preference develops, one can only speculate about how gender dysphoria might lead to autogynephilia. Seil (1996) suggested that, unlike androphilic trans-sexuals, nonandrophilic transsexuals usually experience their cross-gender wishes as ego-dystonic. It is tempting to hypothesize that autogynephilia might develop when ego-dystonic cross-gender feelings somehow interfere with the development of normal erotic interests in other persons. This hypothesis would be consistent with the observation by Blanchard (1992) that auto-gynephilia partially competes with sexual interest in other persons.

CONCLUSIONS

Blanchard's concept of autogynephilia provides a powerful model for understanding the phenomenology of male-to-female transsexualism, and his proposed transsexual typology, which divides transsexuals into androphilic and autogynephilic categories, has considerable heuristic value. But as a practical matter, it is unlikely that many transsexuals who visit mental health professionals will state that their desire to undergo sex reassignment derives primarily from their paraphilic wish to feminize their bodies. Given the stigmatization of anything that appears male-typical in MTF transsexuals, it is remarkable that *any* transsexuals will so state. Yet, clearly there are some applicants for sex reassignment for whom autogynephilic sexual feelings play a prominent, or even central, role. These transsexuals often experience shame and confusion about their autogynephilic feelings, in addition to suffering from gender dysphoria. The concept of autogynephilia can help clinicians to better understand MTF transsexual patients who recognize a strong sexual component to their gender dysphoria. It can also help reassure both patients and caregivers that such feelings are consistent with genuine transsexualism.

REFERENCES

Abel, G.G. & Osborn, C. (1992), The paraphilias. The extent and nature of sexually deviant and criminal behavior. *Psychiat. Clin. North Amer.*, 15:675-687.

Allison, R. (2001), Janice Raymond and autogynephilia. *Transgender Tapestry*, 1(93): 65-67.

American Psychiatric Association (2000), *Diagnostic and Statistical Manual of Mental Disorders (Fourth Edition, Text Revision)*. Washington, DC: Author.

Baker, H.J. (1969), Transsexualism–Problems in treatment. *Amer. J. Psychiat.*, 125: 1412-1418.

Barnes, K. (2001), Some observations on autogynephilia. *Transgender Tapestry*, 1(93):24-25, 62.

Bentler, P.M. (1976), A typology of transsexualism: Gender identity theory and data. *Arch. Sex. Behav.*, 5:567-584.

Blanchard, R. (1985), Typology of male-to-female transsexualism. *Arch. Sex. Behav.*, 14:247-261.

_____ (1987), Heterosexual and homosexual gender dysphoria. *Arch. Sex. Behav.*, 16:139-152.

_____ (1988), Nonhomosexual gender dysphoria. *J. Sex Res.*, 24: 188-193.

_____ (1989a), The classification and labeling of nonhomosexual gender dysphorias. *Arch. Sex. Behav.*, 18:315-334.

_____ (1989b), The concept of autogynephilia and the typology of male gender dysphoria. *J. Nerv. & Ment. Dis.*, 177:616-623.

_____ (1991), Clinical observations and systematic studies of autogynephilia. *J. Sex & Marital Ther.*, 17:235-251.

_____ (1992), Nonmonotonic relation of autogynephilia and heterosexual attraction. *J. Abnorm. Psychol.*, 101:71-276.

_____ (1993a), The she-male phenomenon and the concept of partial autogynephilia. *J. Sex & Mar. Ther.*, 19:69-76.

_____ (1993b), Varieties of autogynephilia and their relationship to gender dysphoria. *Arch. Sex. Behav.*, 22:241-251.

_____ (1993c), Partial versus complete autogynephilia and gender dysphoria. *J. Sex & Marital Ther.*, 19:301-307.

_____ & Clemmensen, L.H. (1988), A test of the *DSM-III-R's* implicit assumption that fetishistic arousal and gender dysphoria are mutually exclusive. *J. Sex Res.*, 25:426-432.

_____, _____ & Steiner, B.W. (1985), Social desirability response set and systematic distortion in the self-report of adult male gender patients. *Arch. Sex. Behav.*, 14:505-516.

_____, _____ & _____ (1987), Heterosexual and homosexual gender dysphoria. *Arch. Sex. Behav.*, 16:139-152.

_____ & Hucker, S.J. (1991), Age, transvestism, bondage, and concurrent paraphilic activities in 117 fatal cases of autoerotic asphyxia. *Brit. J. Psychiat.*, 159:371-377.

_____, Racansky, I.G. & Steiner, B.W. (1986), Phallometric detection of fetishistic arousal in heterosexual male cross-dressers. *J. Sex Res.*, 22:452-462.

_____ & Sheridan, P.M. (1992), Sibship size, sibling sex ratio, birth order, and parental age in homosexual and nonhomosexual gender dysphorics. *J. Nerv. & Ment. Dis.*, 190:40-47.

Buckwalter, L. (2001), Autogynephilia: All dressed up and no one to be. A critique. *Transgender Tapestry*, 1(93):22-23.

Buhrich, N. & McConaghy, N. (1977), Can fetishism occur in transsexuals? *Arch. Sex. Behav.*, 6:223-235.

_____ & _____ (1978), Two clinically discrete syndromes of transsexualism. *Brit. J. Psychiat.*, 133:73-76.

Christie Brown, J.R.W. (1983), Paraphilias: Sadomasochism, fetishism, transvestism, and transsexuality. *Brit. J. Psychiat.*, 143:227-231.

Docter, R.F. (1988), *Transvestites and Transsexuals: Toward a Theory of Cross-gender Behavior.* New York: Plenum.

Doorn, C., Poortinga, J. & Verschoor, A. (1994), Cross-gender identity in transvestites and male transsexuals. *Arch. Sex. Behav.*, 23:185-201.

Freund, K., Steiner, B.W. & Chan, S. (1982), Two types of cross-gender identity. *Arch. Sex. Behav.*, 11:49-63.

Hoenig, J. & Kenna, J.C. (1974), The nosological position of transsexualism. *Arch. Sex. Behav.*, 3:273-287.

Johnson, S. & Hunt, D. (1990), The relationship of male transsexual typology to psychosocial adjustment. *Arch. Sex. Behav.*, 19:349-360.

Kwan, M., Greenleaf, W.J., Mann, J., Crapo, L. & Davidson, J.M. (1983), The nature of androgen action on male sexuality: A combined laboratory-self-report study on hypogonadal men. *J. Clin. Endocrinol. Metab.*, 57:557-562.

Landén, M., Wålinder, J., Hambert, G. & Lundström, B. (1998), Factors predictive of regret in sex reassignment. *Acta Psychiat. Scand.*, 97:284-289.

Langevin, R. (1985), The meanings of cross-dressing. In: *Gender Dysphoria*, ed. B. Steiner. New York: Plenum, pp. 207-225.

Laub, D.R. & Fisk, N.M. (1974), A rehabilitation program for gender dysphoria syndrome by surgical sex change. *Plast. Reconstr. Surg.*, 120:388-403.

Lawrence, A.A. (1998), Men trapped in men's bodies: An introduction to the concept of autogynephilia. *Transgender Tapestry*, 1(85):65-68.

_____ (1999a), 28 narratives about autogynephilia. Retrieved April 25, 2003, from <http://www.annelawrence.com/agnarratives.html>.

_____ (1999b), 31 new narratives about autogynephilia. Retrieved April 25, 2003, from <http://www.annelawrence.com/31narratives.html>.

_____ (1999c), Lessons from autogynephiles: Eroticism, motivation, and the Standards of Care. Paper presented at the Harry Benjamin International Gender Dysphoria Association XVI Biennial Symposium, London.

_____ (2000), Sexuality and transsexuality: A new introduction to autogynephilia. *Transgender Tapestry*, 1(92):17-23.

_____ (2003), Factors associated with satisfaction or regret following male-to-female sex reassignment surgery. *Arch. Sex. Behav.*, 32:299-315.

_____ (unpublished paper), Sexuality before and after male-to-female sex reassignment surgery.

Leavitt, F. & Berger, J.C. (1990), Clinical patterns among male transsexual candidates with erotic interest in males. *Arch. Sex. Behav.*, 19:491-505.

Levine, S.B. (1993), Gender-disturbed males. *J. Sex & Marital Ther.*, 19:131-141.

_____, Risen, C.B. & Althof, S.E. (1990), Essay on the diagnosis and nature of paraphilia. *J. Sex & Marital Ther.*, 16:89-102.

Lundström, B., Pauly, I. & Wålinder, J. (1984), Outcomes of sex reassignment surgery. *Acta Psychiat. Scand.*, 70:289-294.

Masters, W.H. & Johnson, V.E. (1966), *Human Sexual Response*. Boston: Little, Brown.

Meyer, J.K. (1982), The theory of the gender identity disorders. *J. Amer. Psychoanal. Assn.*, 30:381-418.

Muirhead-Allwood, S.K., Royle, M.G. & Young, R. (1999), Sexuality and satisfaction with surgical results in male-to-female transsexuals. Poster session presented at the Harry Benjamin International Gender Dysphoria Association XVI Biennial Symposium, London.

Seil, D. (1996), Transsexuals: The boundary of sexual identity and gender. In: *Textbook of Homosexuality and Mental Health*, eds. R.P. Cabaj & T.S. Stein. Washington, DC: American Psychiatric Press, pp. 743-762.

Sørensen, T. (1981), A follow-up study of operated transsexual males. *Acta Psychiat. Scand.*, 63:486-503.

Stoller, R.J. (1985), *Presentations of Gender*. New Haven, CT: Yale University Press.

Wilson, G.D. & Gosselin, C. (1980), Personality characteristics of fetishists, transvestites, and masochists. *Pers. Individ. Dif.*, 1:289-295.

Zucker, K.J & Blanchard, R. (1997), Transvestic fetishism: Psychopathology and theory. In: *Sexual Deviance*, eds. D.R. Laws & W. O'Donohue. New York: Plenum, pp. 253-279.

"Qué joto bonita!":
Transgender Negotiations
of Sex and Ethnicity

Vernon A. Rosario, MD, PhD

SUMMARY. Recent transgender literature has been sharply critical of existing medical models of the psychosexual development of transsexuals and of the treatment of Gender Identity Disorder. Transgender authors have pointed out that subjects have deliberately falsified their reports in order to conform to medical and psychiatric models for the sake of gaining access to services. In newer transsexual narratives, gender and sexual orientation development appear far more fluid and ambiguous over the life span.

This paper reviews the nosological history of gender atypicality, from nineteenth century "sexual inversion" to transvestitism and transsexualism, examining how deviations of gender identity, gender role, sexual object, and sexual aim were often collapsed together. These imbrications continue to persist in both the medical and popular literature on transsexualism.

A topic that has especially been neglected is the relationship of ethnicity to the development of gender and sexual identity. Presented is case material gathered from dynamic psychotherapy with a Latina, trans-

Vernon A. Rosario is Clinical Instructor, University of California–Los Angeles Neuropsychiatric Institute.

Address correspondence to: Vernon A. Rosario, MD, PhD, 10850 Wilshire Boulevard, Suite 1210, Los Angeles, CA 90024 (E-mail: vrosario@post.harvard.edu).

[Haworth co-indexing entry note]: ""Qué joto bonita!": Transgender Negotiations of Sex and Ethnicity." Rosario, Vernon A. Co-published simultaneously in *Journal of Gay & Lesbian Psychotherapy* (The Haworth Medical Press, an imprint of The Haworth Press, Inc.) Vol. 8, No. 1/2, 2004, pp. 89-97; and: *Transgender Subjectivities: A Clinician's Guide* (ed: Ubaldo Leli, and Jack Drescher) The Haworth Medical Press, an imprint of The Haworth Press, Inc., 2004, pp. 89-97. Single or multiple copies of this article are available for a fee from The Haworth Document Delivery Service [1-800-HAWORTH, 9:00 a.m. - 5:00 p.m. (EST). E-mail address: docdelivery@haworthpress.com].

gendered sex worker which illustrates the articulations of ethnicity, gender, and sexuality in both the transgendered subject and her heterosexually-identified male partners. *[Article copies available for a fee from The Haworth Document Delivery Service: 1-800-HAWORTH. E-mail address: <docdelivery@haworthpress.com> Website: <http://www.HaworthPress.com> © 2004 by The Haworth Press, Inc. All rights reserved.]*

KEYWORDS. Cross-dressing, ethnicity, gender dysphoria, gender identity disorder, GID, homosexuality, Latina, Latino, psychotherapy, sex reassignment, she-male, transgender, transsexual, transvestivism, vestida

THEORETICAL ORIENTATION

From the outset, I should say that my perspective avoids seeing transsexualism or transgenderism as pathological or as a disorder in itself, but as "normal"–albeit a rare form of normality–in other words, a natural variant of human sexuality. If we take this approach, how can it affect our understanding of gender and sexuality more generally? Can transgenderism even help us explain heterosexuality and conventional gender identity? Here, Freud's comment on the mysteries of homosexuality and heterosexuality remain just as true today. In the "Three Essays on the Theory of Sexuality," Freud wrote:

> Psycho-analytic research is most decidedly opposed to any attempt at separating off homosexuals from the rest of mankind as a group of a special character . . . [F]rom the point of view of psycho-analysis the exclusive sexual interest felt by men for women is also a problem that needs elucidating and is not a self-evident fact based upon an attraction that is ultimately of a chemical nature. (Freud, 1905, p. 145)

The neurobiology and the developmental history of heterosexuality remain just as mysterious as that of homosexuality or transsexualism, perhaps even more so, since most people think of heterosexuality as not needing an explanation and just happening in the natural course of things. Transgendered individuals, as they self-consciously negotiate the vicissitudes of erotic and gendered life, can help us gain a different perspective on gender and sexual development.

HISTORICAL REVIEW

For a century, transsexuals have been masked by their medical construction (King, 1987). The 19th and early 20th century medical literature includes many clinical case studies that, in retrospect, we might identify as manifestations of transsexualism. Patients described themselves as being female souls trapped in a male body or vice versa. But at the time these were labeled as cases of "sexual inversion" which later became synonymous with "homosexuality." Felix Abraham (1931) labeled as "homosexual transvestites" the two patients upon whom he performed the first "genital transformation" (*Genitalumwandlung*) surgery in 1931. Likewise, the diagnosis of "genuine transvestitism" was applied to Christine Jorgensen, whose surgical sex change drew enormous media attention in 1953 (Hamburger, Stürup, and Dahl-Iversen 1953; Meyerowitz, 1998). That same year, at the Symposium on Transsexualism and Transvestitism, its organizer, endocrinologist Harry Benjamin, presented transsexualism as the "extreme degree of transvestitism" (1954). Although the term "transsexual" was coined by Magnus Hirschfeld in 1923 (in an article on "intersexuals"), it did not gain widespread usage until it was used in 1949 by David O. Cauldwell in describing a case of severe gender dysphoria (Hirschfeld, 1923; Cauldwell, 1949).

The psychiatric model that evolved in the 1950s viewed transsexualism as a mental illness that, uniquely, could be treated with a combination of psychological, hormonal, and surgical interventions. In 1979, The Harry Benjamin International Dysphoria Association proposed standards of care for gender identity disorders (GID); these have been revised five times since then. These required a sequence of real-life passing (originally one year, now reduced to three months), at least one year of hormone therapy and passing, and finally surgical genital and breast reconstruction. Through a complete course of sex reassignment, transsexualism could be cured, erased. The patients were usually encouraged to delete their past lives, move to a new town, and start up again as a "normal" male or female. For decades, then, transsexualism was a liminal and pathologized subject position frequently conflated with homosexuality and transvestitism.

According to this medical model, transsexualism had an infantile onset in effeminate boys or tomboy girls, and a lifelong sense of gender difference turning to dysphoria. The ideal, successfully treated transsexuals underwent full gender transition, becoming heterosexual and exhibiting stereotypical gender roles. However, as was already becoming evident in Garfinkel's discussion of "Agnes" (a male-to-female transsexual patient treated at UCLA by Robert Stoller) patients were deceiving their doctors (Garfinkel, 1967). Patients had read the medical literature, knew the medical model, and parroted this back in order to gain access to hormonal and surgical treatment.

THE EMERGENCE OF TRANSSEXUALISM

In the past decade, transsexuals have come out of the closet and been more honest about the complexity of their erotic and gender experiences and desires. A new line of transgender theory has been developing in print, at conferences, and on the World Wide Web, thanks to transgender academic and community theorists. The Web especially is becoming the major means of exchanging information (including tips on hormone self-dosing and home breast enlargement).

The Web has also exploded with sites catering to those erotically interested in transsexuals. "Transgenderism" has, therefore, become the current umbrella term to include a diversity of unorthodox gender positions, roles, or explorations including: transsexualism under the old medical model; transvestitism; part-time passing; androgyny or gender-fuck; and passing with few or no hormonal or surgical interventions ("nontransitioning transsexuals"). The distinction between transsexual and transgender is a highly policed one, and to some extent falls along generational lines. Older transsexuals, particularly male-to-females who have undergone full sex reassignment surgery (SRS), often view younger transgender individuals who do not want SRS as fence sitters who are not "real" transsexuals, just gender dabblers. Elkins and King (1997) describe the phenomenon as "gender blending."

Transgender theorists informed by feminist and queer theory have been especially critical of the biomedical constructions of transgenderism, the phallocentrism of medicine (particularly surgery), and gender normativeness in psychiatry. The very notion of GID has been much debated. Some activists argue for its elimination from the *Diagnostic and Statistical Manual of Mental Disorders (DSM)* in the same way that homosexuality and ego-dystonic homosexuality were eliminated in the 1970s and 1980s, respectively. Others see GID as a necessary evil for justifying insurance coverage of medical services.

Apart from the critique of medicine, transgender individuals have explored and expanded on the stereotypical models of transsexuality. Sandy Stone's "Post-Transsexual Manifesto" (1991) was a rallying call to transsexuals to deliver honest autobiographical narratives that challenge or even subvert the model of passing. These newer transgender narratives point out a far more complex relationship between gender identity and orientation. Newer transgender stories now acknowledge a later onset of gender questioning, exploration, and fluidity. Sexual orientation often also becomes a part of this exploration, whether during the time of gender questioning or after sex reassignment.

Another aspect of this efflorescence of transgenderism is the decentralization of treatment away from a handful of academic centers to outpatient clinics. Hysterectomies are increasingly being performed by transgender-sympathetic gynecologists not as SRS, but as the treatment for severe dysmenorrhea. Breast surgeries are more available as elective, cosmetic procedures in the US and in Mexico, creating "she-males."

She-males are individuals with a penis and varying degrees of hormonal or surgical breast enlargement, who largely pass as women. The "she-male phenomenon" was first described in the medical literature in 1993 under the label of "partial autogynephilia" (Blanchard, 1993). As for those who love them, they have been given the awkward but scientifically reifying label of "gynandromorphophiles" (Blanchard and Collins, 1993). A new market has cropped up around she-males, with magazines like *Transformation* catering to them and those who desire them. There are even transsexual sex toys, and a proliferation of she-male porn videos.

What has not been examined much in this new literature is the role of ethnicity. Third Wave feminism undermined the notion of a universal or uniform female identity or "women's experience" by analyzing how race, ethnicity, and class significantly color gender. I feel it is necessary now to examine the articulations of transgenderism and ethnicity–as demonstrated in the following case study/psychoethnography of a patient I saw for psychotherapy for a year.

CASE STUDY: FRANCES

Frances is a 39-year-old Mexican-American, who presents herself in the clinic in casual, loose-fitting clothes. Although she is very slight and pretty, and could easily pass as a woman, she uses makeup only occasionally and sparingly, and generally appears androgynous.

Frances was born and raised in San Diego, and is the eldest of three children, with a brother a year younger and a sister 2 years junior. Her father is a military man who was very strict, terse, and cold. Her mother is a homemaker whom Frances describes as emotional, loving, and close. She reports having been a quiet, introverted child with crushes only on boys since age 9, but no real sense of gender or sexual difference per se. At age 12, he began having an erotic interest in boys and began developing an identity as a gay man. He was also increasingly teased by his peers and chastised by his father for being a "sissy." His first romantic involvement was with a classmate at age 15. All hell broke loose when his mother discovered their love letters, and prohibited the two boys from seeing each other. The word of their affair spread at school: he was further taunted and his boyfriend avoided him entirely. (The boyfriend, Frances later learned, had married and become a father.) His parents forced him to see a psychiatrist–who, fortunately, did not pathologize his behavior. At this time, Frances began suffering from severe, recurrent depression and made his first suicide attempt by overdosing on his mother's medicines. He dropped out of school.

At age 19 he met a cultured, somewhat effeminate gay man, 5 years Frances's senior, who became his boyfriend for 9 years. They lived together and socialized as a gay couple. However, Frances never felt that he totally fit into the gay identity. He never felt comfortable sexually: he avoided using his penis and never ejaculated when having sex with his boyfriend. Instead he preferred, then and now, to masturbate alone when he was really horny, and felt that he had to "get the testosterone out of [his] system." He completed his high school equivalency diploma and earned a college degree in art. He dreamed of becoming a painter. She recalls this as her "Boy George phase," when he dressed flamboyantly and wanted to stand out. He was out to his family as a gay man. His mother accepted his homosexuality, although she made it clear she would prefer him to be straight, marry, and have children. His father never wanted to discuss it.

When he broke up with his boyfriend, he moved to Los Angeles and began working in a corporate trading firm. It was a very straight environment. He also began hanging out at Latino gay clubs all of which featured elaborately choreographed drag shows and lip-synched impersonations of Latina singers. The original female singers, with their hyperfeminine, dramatic style, already seem to be imitating drag performances. Frances began socializing with the drag artists. He began exploring cross-dressing at night while dressing in a business suit by day. But he was increasingly overwhelmed by the yoke of a tie. He gradually began acknowledging a transgender identity in his early 30s, and started hormone therapy.

For the past eight years she has worked in the sex trade as a she-male. Her escort ad reads: "I'd love to be your wife tonight, let's play house. I pack 8 functional inches in my panties." The emphasis on the penis is central to the phallic appeal of the she-male. Frances jokes that with the hormones it isn't 8 inches any more and never becomes erect with her "johns," but they all want her to hike up her dress and show off her penis. She notes that most of them are straight-identified men, many of them married. She feels most of them are "closet cases," i.e., they are not out as she-male lovers. They report similar stories of having encountered a she-male prostitute by accident once and ever since then became hooked. They love gazing, playing, sucking her penis while they masturbate. "It's crazy," she says, "They pay me $100 to suck *my* dick." While early on she took all comers, she is now more selective. She avoids anyone with an accent–primarily Latinos. She finds the white men tend to be married, guilt-ridden, speedy, and more generous. The Latino guys are too rough, want to use drugs, come in groups, do not appreciate her humor, and are miserly. She has also noticed increasingly younger guys, in their early 20s, soliciting her and already being quite focused in their erotic desires for she-males.

Her search for a partner is equally selective. Her erotic ideal would be a hot, sweaty, super-masculine, straight, white guy, because they make her feel more feminine. Yet she also deeply yearns for someone intellectually and artistically compatible. Last year she placed an ad in an HIV-positive personals column, advertising herself as an androgynous, "cool, modern, HIV + dreamer."

Through the ad she met a straight-identified, Italian-American man, whose previous girlfriend was also a she-male. They dated for several months before moving in together. She likes him because he is such a "masculine, regular Joe" and he loves her feminine looks. However, he is uncomfortable with her being boyish and is not emotionally supportive. They recently broke up after he hit her, precipitating a depressive tailspin, and another suicide attempt.

She still feels as if she is going through a chaotic period of gender construction. She sees herself alternating between two positions: a shy, weak boy, and a strong, mature woman. She regrets that as she becomes more of a woman, she has to leave the boy behind, and she feels divided, like a freak at times. And it's when people (usually heterosexuals) regard her as a freak that she is most wounded. Nevertheless, like other transgendered individuals, she currently prefers the ambiguous position and is not interested in full SRS. She likes being confused for a cute gay man or spotted as transgendered: hence she was pleased with the catcall, "*Qué joto bonita!*" from some Latino construction workers.

She has very limited contact with her parents. She has explained to them that she is undergoing hormone therapy and now prefers to be referred to as a female. Her father refuses to acknowledge her gender change and continues to criticize her effeminate presentation. Her mother, on the other hand, while still mystified by the changes, wrote Frances a letter in December 1998 blessing her SRS.

CONCLUSIONS

Let me stop here and draw up some observations–albeit very tentative, given that I worked only briefly with Frances. Her case, nevertheless, highlights how, unlike models of transsexualism developed in the 1950s and 60s, transgenderism is not experienced or related as a linear narrative of sex switching to conform to congenital, fixed, ontologically authentic gender. This model is still dominant among many transsexuals (particularly older ones), who support genetic and neurobiological theories of transsexualism (Kirk, 1999; Norton, 1999). The evolution of Frances's gender identity and sexuality has taken many twists and turns, and is still sensed as "work in progress." She sees neither hormones nor surgery as a solution or a cure.

Her Mexican-American ethnicity also clearly shapes her notions of gender and sexuality–in terms of ideals and roles to be imitated or resisted. The differences in acculturation between her and her parents also pose challenges to being understood and accepted by them. Yet the high value of the family drives her mother's sustained attachment and support (however uneasy). Frances's selection of sexual partners and clients is strongly directed by ethnicity and class, as these are culturally associated with differences in masculinity, aggressivity, and sexual orientation.

It is not necessarily ego-dystonic for a straight-identified Latino man to have sex as an active, penetrative "top" with effeminate men or transsexuals. As Prieur suggests in, *Mema's House* (1998), her ethnography of a community of working-class *vestidas* (male-to-female transgenders) in Mexico City, a man is a man as long as he remains impenetrable. A similar dynamic has been described in other cultures with strictly differentiated gender roles, as well as in the United States in the early 20th century and, still currently, in working class populations (Balderston and Guy, 1997; Murray and Roscoe, 1997; Green, 1999; Chauncey, 1994).

While this gender rigidity can contribute to hostility and even violence toward gender-unconventional people (as was the case with Brandon Teena as rendered in the movie *Boys Don't Cry*), the machista system of dichotomized gender roles also legitimizes special niches for transgenders: as drag performers or she-male sex workers, for example. However, we should also keep in mind that this dichotomized system is historically and culturally dynamic, since the commodification of the she-male has only occurred to a significant degree in the past decade.

Finally, I do not want to neglect or minimize the mental health problems of Frances and other transgendered individuals. Her mood disorder and characterological problems are certainly not independent of her gender and sexuality concerns; however, I choose not to interpret them as *caused* by her transgenderism. As with all of us, mental health is interwoven with the complex historical and cultural tapestry that constitutes gender, ethnicity, and sexuality. Teasing at the well-knotted threads of that tapestry in a personal probing and subversion is a courageous act, that is, not surprisingly, psychologically demanding. Given the hostile reception that most transgendered individuals have received from family, society, and medical providers, it is essential that mental health professionals provide a sympathetic and safe space for exploration. And it is particularly important a sensitive cultural perspective be brought to that exploration.

REFERENCES

Abraham, F. (1931), Genitalumwandlungen an zwei männlichen Transvestiten. *Zeitschrift für Sexualwissenschaft und Sexualpolitik*, 18:223-226.

Balderston, D. & Guy, D., eds. (1997), *Sex and Sexuality in Latin America*. New York: New York University Press.

Benjamin, H. (1954), Transsexualism and transvestitism as psychosomatic and somato-psychic syndromes. *Amer. J. Psychother.*, 8:219-239.

_____ (1966), *The Transsexual Phenomenon*. New York: Julian Press.

Blanchard, R. (1993), The she-male phenomenon and the concept of partial auto-gynephilia. *J. Sex & Marital Ther.,* 19:69-76.

_____ & Collins, P. (1993), Men with sexual interest in transvestites, transsexuals, and she-males. *J. Nerv. & Ment. Disease,* 181:570-5.

Cauldwell, D. (1949), Psychopathia transsexuals. *Sexology,* 16:274-280.

Chauncey, G. (1994). *Gay New York: Gender, Urban Culture and the Making of the Gay Male World, 1890-1940.* New York: Basic Books.

Elkins, R. & King, D. (1997), Blending genders: Contributions to the emerging field of transgender studies. *IJT,* 1:1.

Freud, S. (1905), Three essays on the theory of sexuality. *Standard Edition,* 7: 145-146n. London: Hogarth Press, 1953.

Garfinkel, H. (1967), *Studies in Ethnomethodology.* Englewood Cliffs, NJ: Prentice Hall.

Green, J. (1999), *Beyond Carnival: Male Homosexuality in Twentieth-Century Brazil.* Chicago: University of Chicago Press.

Hamburger, C., Stürup, G.K. & Dahl-Iversen, E. (1953), Transvestism: hormonal, psychiatric, and surgical treatment. *J. Am. Med. Assoc.,* 152:391-396.

Herdt, G., ed. (1994), *Third Sex, Third Gender: Beyond Sexual Dimorphism in Culture and History.* New York: Zone Books.

Hirschfeld, M. (1910), *Die Transvestiten. Eine Untersuchung über den erotischen Verkleidungstrieb mit umfangreichem casuistischem und historischen Material, Vol I-II.* Berlin: Alfred Pulvermacher.

_____ (1923), Die intersexuelle Konstitution. *Jahrbuch für sexuelle Zwischenstufen,* 23:3-27.

King, D. (1987), Social constructionism and medical knowledge: The case of trans-sexualism. *Sociology of Health & Illness,* 9:351-77.

Kirk, S. (1999), The Brain: A brief look at our nervous system. *Transgender Comm. News,* 9:16-17.

Meyerowitz, J. (1998), Sex-change and the popular press: Historical notes on trans-sexuality in the United States, 1930-1955. *GLQ* 4:159-87.

Murray, S. & Roscoe,W., eds. (1997), *Islamic Homosexualities: Culture, History, and Literature.* New York: New York University Press.

Norton, J. (1999), "You are a very beautiful woman, even though you are a man": The vestidas of Mexico City [book review of Prieur 1998]. *Transgen. Tap.,* 88:40.

Prieur, A. (1998), *Mema's House, Mexico City: On Transvestites, Queens, and Machos.* Chicago: University of Chicago Press.

Stoller, R. (1975), *Sex and Gender, Vol. II: The Transsexual Experiment.* New York: Jason Aronson.

Stone, S. (1991), The Empire strikes back: A post-transsexual manifesto. In: *Body Guards: The Cultural Politics of Gender Ambiguity,* eds. J. Epstein & K. Straub. New York: Routledge, pp. 280-304.

The Diagnosis and Treatment of Transgendered Patients

David Seil, MD

SUMMARY. The diagnosis and treatment of 271 transgendered patients is described. Characteristics of the transgendered patients seen by the author between 1979 and 2001 reveal four distinct groups not specified in the current *Diagnostic and Statistical Manual (DSM-IV)* description. These characteristics are important because they determine the internal and external difficulties the patients present to the clinician. Statistics on age, gender, relationships, occupation, education, drug/alcohol abuse, secondary diagnoses and sexual orientation of each subgroup are presented and discussed. *[Article copies available for a fee from The Haworth Document Delivery Service: 1-800-HAWORTH. E-mail address: <docdelivery@ haworthpress.com> Website: <http://www.HaworthPress.com> © 2004 by The Haworth Press, Inc. All rights reserved.]*

KEYWORDS. Cross-dressing, *Diagnostic and Statistical Manual*, gender dysphoria, gender identity, gender identity disorder, GID, mood disorder, sex reassignment, transgender, transsexual

---

David Seil is a psychiatrist, now retired, previously in private practice in Boston, MA.

Address correspondence to: David Seil, MD, 2508 Monterey Street, Sarasota, FL 34231 (E-mail: Davids2189@aol.com).

[Haworth co-indexing entry note]: "The Diagnosis and Treatment of Transgendered Patients." Seil, David. Co-published simultaneously in *Journal of Gay & Lesbian Psychotherapy* (The Haworth Medical Press, an imprint of The Haworth Press, Inc.) Vol. 8, No. 1/2, 2004, pp. 99-116; and: *Transgender Subjectivities: A Clinician's Guide* (ed: Ubaldo Leli, and Jack Drescher) The Haworth Medical Press, an imprint of The Haworth Press, Inc., 2004, pp. 99-116. Single or multiple copies of this article are available for a fee from The Haworth Document Delivery Service [1-800-HAWORTH, 9:00 a.m. - 5:00 p.m. (EST). E-mail address: docdelivery@haworthpress.com].

INTRODUCTION

Clinical observation of 271 transgendered patients seen by the author between 1979 and June 2001 reveals four separate subgroups not specified in the *Diagnostic and Statistical Manual (DSM-IV)*. These patients have been seen for evaluation and in some cases ongoing treatment.

Gender Identity Disorder (GID) is defined in *DSM-IV* (American Psychiatric Association, 1994, pp. 532-538) as follows:

A. A strong and persistent cross-gender identification manifested by symptoms such as a stated desire to be the other sex, frequent passing as the other sex, desire to live or be treated as the other sex, or the conviction that he or she has the typical feelings and reactions of the other sex.
B. Persistent discomfort with his or her sex or sense of inappropriateness in the gender role of that sex . . . manifested by symptoms such as preoccupation with getting rid of primary and secondary sex characteristics . . . or belief that he or she was born the wrong sex.
C. The disturbance is not concurrent with a physical intersex condition.
D. The condition causes clinically significant distress or impairment in social, occupational, or other important areas of functioning.

GID is a rare condition. The incidence of GID as reported in *DSM-IV* (American Psychiatric Association, 1994, p. 535) is 1:30,000 for natal males, 1:100,000 for natal females. Interestingly, in The Netherlands, the incidence reported in 1988 as 1:18,000 for natal males and 1:54,000 for natal females. By 1990, the incidence for natal males had increased to 1:11,900, and the incidence for natal females remained the same (Bakker et al., 1993). This disparity between the US estimate and the Dutch estimate may be attributed to the favorable climate for acceptance and treatment in The Netherlands. The prevalence in Singapore is even higher (Bakker et al., 1993). Most likely, because therapeutic services for GID are scarce in this country, the prevalence here is underestimated. The ratio of transgendered men to women remains at approximately 3:1 in both countries.

TERMINOLOGY

Since this paper presents material regarding sex, gender, and gender roles, clarification of terms is essential for understanding the complex nature of GID. In the *DSM-IV* description, "sex" refers to both *anatomic* and *genetic gender* and does so interchangeably. The genetic sex or gender is assumed to be either XX or XY, and since chromosomal studies are not done on the majority of patients, this assumption cannot be challenged at present. Anatomic configuration is used most frequently to assign male or female at birth and is assumed to match chromosomal gender. There can be a distinction between *genetic gender* and *anatomic gender.* In this paper, references to male or female refer to the gender that was assigned at birth, i.e., *natal male* or *natal female,* even though this type of gender assignment ignores conditions in which genital configuration does not follow chromosomal gender. *Gender role* is an important concept in respect to the behaviors that are mentioned as indicative of GID. The *DSM-IV* criteria follow the western concept of dichotomous or binary gender-appropriate roles and behavior. Society endorses certain gender roles as being appropriate. Subsequent gender-specific behaviors are expected quickly after gender assignment occurs, and if the genetic sex of the child is known prenatally through amniocentesis, these expectations can begin even before birth.

GID vividly illustrates that another factor unknown at birth plays an important role in the later life of the child. This is *gender identity.* Gender identity is the subjective sense of the gender one feels one is, regardless of what genitals a person has. If the genitals are male, and the gender identification is male, the individual comfortably selects what roles are appropriate and usually enjoys being male and meeting male obligations and doing socially approved male things that suit his personality, be it chess or football. Obviously the obverse is true for the female. However, germane to this paper, there are those for whom the internal gender identity does not match the natal sex, and for them, as is shown below, the socially appropriate gender roles are not comfortable. The discomfort that results regarding one's assigned gender is called *gender dysphoria.* If gender dysphoria is persistent, and the individual desires to live in the other gender, this individual suffers from GID.

The terms transsexual and transsexuality have largely fallen out of use with the community of transgendered people and the clinicians involved in treating them. *DSM III-R* (American Psychiatric Association, 1987, pp. 74-76) labeled GID as "Transsexualism," which approached creating a third gender category. Nevertheless, a basic concept in that diagnostic description still remains: individuals with GID do not wish to be considered another category of gender. Most of them deeply desire to move from one conventional gender to the other. They adopt not only the anatomy of the other gender but also enter into roles determined by society as appropriate to the other gender. In doing so, as the disorder disappears, they disappear into the fabric of society.

DIAGNOSIS

How is GID diagnosed? Observation that an individual displays behaviors that cross the boundaries of traditionally accepted gender role behavior cannot be used as the sole indicator that an individual wishes to make a gender shift. Behaviors in this area change as fashions and social mores change. For example, earrings on men are no longer viewed as designating femininity, no more so than a reversal of traditional roles for a heterosexual couple (woman working, man staying home to care for children) would signify a gender identity crossover. On the other hand, occasional cross-dressing that does not qualify as a "persistent" role exchange necessary to meet the criteria for the diagnosis of GID may signify an underlying gender disorder. Pre-transition men and women with GID will occasionally cross-dress, often in secret, because such activity provides great pleasure and relief from the distress of GID. Conversely, the transgendered individual who has an ego-dystonic opposite gender identity often behaves in an overdetermined masculine or feminine manner with such success that it is a shock to his or her intimates when the inner identity is revealed. The observer has seen nothing in their role behaviors to give any clue that a gender conflict existed. Thus the diagnosis of GID cannot be made by observation of behavior:

> When A. called for an appointment, she stated that she had chosen to see me because of my expertise in gender identity. She appeared in the office as a late middle-aged woman somewhat mannish in dress and manner. I stated that I assumed she wished to talk about transitioning to male. Obviously surprised, A. stated, "Doctor, I am an XY! I had my surgery thirty-five years ago." A. sought treatment for chronic depression and chose someone with knowledge of GID because she did not want that to be the issue.

GID is a diagnosis made by self-reportage, and the only means by which to diagnose GID is by listening to the patient. This presented some problems for many clinicians who were early workers in this field. Since so many of the patients told the same story, the clinicians became suspicious that the applicants for treatment were being coached in order to obtain surgeries. What the clinicians did not realize was that the course of GID varies little in substance from one person to another within each subgroup of patients. At the same time, these clinicians were strongly invested in creating stereotypically "normal" men and women.

> *"What chance does this forty-six year old man have of ever looking like a woman?"* (from an independent evaluation done on an early patient of the author's)

Appearance–ability to "pass" as a member of the new gender–was of great concern to these clinicians, at times even more so than to their patients. The caregivers had definite preconceived ideas as to how a man or woman should look and act. Although passing is of great concern to many individuals with GID, it is no longer a major concern to most clinicians.

GENERAL TREATMENT PROTOCOL

GID is a biopsychosocial disorder requiring the intervention of a team of professionals from general medicine, endocrinology, surgery, psychiatry, psychology, and social work. A general protocol for the treatment of GID has been developed by the Harry Benjamin International Gender Dysphoria Association (HBIGDA).[1] HBIGDA is a group of several hundred multidisciplinary caregivers worldwide who provide care to gender dysphoric people. This protocol, called *The Standards of Care (SOC)* (Meyer et al., 2001), outlines timely steps in treatment that include sexual surgeries and psychotherapy. For natal males, treatment begins with a three-month evaluation by an experienced therapist in order to verify the diagnosis of GID and readiness to begin transition. At the end of that time, feminizing hormone therapy can be recommended. The administration of estrogen compounds and testosterone blockers to a male results in the development of mammary glandular tissue, loss of muscle, redistribution of fatty tissue and softening of the skin. Hair loss is stopped, and beard and body hair growth slowed. However, the voice does not rise, and lost head hair does not grow back. Before these changes are noticeable, the individual experiences subjective changes in mood, libido and attitude.

Personal satisfaction with the subjective changes is taken as a positive diagnostic sign in the *SOC*. When the patient is ready, he begins what is called the life test–living as a woman in all areas of life. At the end of one year, sexual reassignment surgery can be recommended by the therapist with a supporting second-opinion. One of the two recommendations needs to be made by a doctoral-level professional mental health specialist. Verification of appropriate medical and endocrinologic treatment must also be provided. Natal males also need to undergo whatever electrolysis or laser treatments are necessary to remove facial and body hair. These patients may also elect other cosmetic procedures to reduce male appearance and promote female persona, but such surgeries are considered a personal, not a clinical decision.

For natal females, the same period of psychological evaluation is necessary before the administration of testosterone. Testosterone stops menses, increases muscle mass and libido, and eventually stimulates baldness, body and facial hair growth, voice lowering and acne. As with the natal males above, personal satisfaction with increased libido and aggressiveness is taken as a positive diagnostic sign in the *SOC*. As their bodies begin to masculinize, bilateral mastectomy is desirable, and two separate recommendations are needed before this procedure is performed. The general thinking within HBIGDA is that it is not feasible for a natal female to successfully complete a yearlong life test as a male before mastectomy. However, since the procedure is financially not available to all, many females-to-males do successfully live as males without mastectomy. Penile constructive surgeries are regarded as not fully successful, and many chose to postpone them. With testosterone, the clitoris can increase to a length permitting vaginal insertion. Complete hysterectomy becomes a matter of choice and availability, as well.

Although the *SOC* are generally followed, exceptions can be made under the right circumstances, as the following vignette shows:

> K. presented as a fifty-year-old woman. In fact she was a natal male who had been living as a female since the age of sixteen when she ran away from home. After a brief period of adolescent prostitution, she took some secretarial courses and began to work in the administration of a civic entity. With altered documents, she had entered into two legal marriages in which her husbands knew of her situation. She lived as a working middle-class wife in a childless marriage. She had not had hormones consistently. Her employer changed the organization health plan to an HMO, and when K. told her story to her new female primary care physician, the physician set into motion the necessary paper work to obtain hormone therapy and sexual reassignment surgery for K. as quickly as possible. Since K. had lived all of her adult life as a woman and had no secondary psychiatric diagnosis, it was decided to waive the *SOC*. K. was enormously relieved to finally be anatomically female. "I could not let either of my husbands touch me below the waist."

K's story is unusual. Few can hide a secret of this magnitude so well for so long.

Part D of the *DSM-IV* criteria addresses the basic definition of a disorder, i.e., a condition that causes severe distress or dysfunction in an important area of living, referring to the psychosocial issues in GID. While the medical treatments that are necessary in order to change the physical attributes of the individual as far as possible towards the other gender are clear and straightforward, the psychosocial issues are by far more complex. It is in this area that the work of the psychotherapist is most essential.

Two treatment issues raised by many transgendered patients need to be mentioned. The first issue is helping the patient move away from rigid social stereotypes and towards the realization that men and women show enormous variation in behavior and physical presentation. The most successful "passing" begins when the internal identity becomes the engine for the mechanics of gender expression regardless of appearance.

Sexual orientation is the second issue that many transgendered patients face. Early candidates had difficulty obtaining surgery if they could not say that post-surgically they would be heterosexual. Because the clinicians were determined to have their patients lead "normal" lives, men and women who knew they would be homosexual following transition were disqualified as candidates for surgery. Since many of them knew this ahead of time, they did indeed prevaricate regarding that aspect of themselves. When the statistics regarding sexual orientation for transgendered individuals are seen, this obviously was an issue for many of them. While it is no longer a problem in obtaining surgery, orientation is a personal issue for the transgendered individual, who may not know what his or her orientation will be until after surgery.

RESULTS

While the general treatment protocol is detailed in the *SOC*, some treatment issues are specific to each subgroup. Before exploring these specific issues, it is helpful to see the demographics of each group. In GID, the particular distress or dysfunction the person experiences depends on the individual's developmental history. Review of these developmental histories reveals four distinct groups that represent different sets of issues. The first distinction that can be made within the total sample is to which gender the person has been natally assigned, male or female. Male or female means that the person has primary and secondary sex characteristics of one or the other and has been raised with synchronous male or female role expectations. The males form a group that desires a physical and social change to female: male-to-female (MTF). Analogously, the females desire a change to male: female-to-male (FTM). Since, as previously stated, gender assignment has been made mostly by visual inspection and not chromosomal analysis, it can only be assumed whether these people are XY or XX. The first division of the sample is thus into MTF or FTM, based on natal gender.

Subsequently, each group can be divided into two subgroups, unofficially labeled *primary* and *secondary*. The primary groups include those transgendered individuals who are aware of their internal cross-gendered identity from an early age and are not conflicted about feeling this way.

C. entered treatment in order to begin hormone therapy. The 26-year-old assigned male presented as female in manner, expression and dress. She had been born with ambiguous genitalia and had undergone over twenty surgeries before puberty to produce male genitalia. Through these ordeals, she had firmly insisted that she was really a girl. Chromosomal studies revealed that she was XXY. Since adolescence, in order to validate her femaleness, she had been promiscuous with men. Estrogens were started, but C. was HIV+, and became too ill to remain in treatment.

For C., her internal identity as a female was ego-syntonic. She was completely comfortable with it, and no amount of surgery or social pressure changed that. These men and women are MTF ego-syntonic, or MTF primary (MTFP), and FTM ego-syntonic or FTM primary (FTMP).

Another group of patients experience quite a different situation. Early awareness of transgendered feelings brought internal discomfort because these feelings were in conflict with other parts of their psychic structure, usually internalized parental/social attitudes. In other words, these feelings became and remained ego-dystonic and thus were not integrated into the personality. These patients would be called MTF ego-dystonic and FTM ego-dystonic. The modifier "secondary" has also been applied here (MTFS and FTMS). The author's sample has been broken down according to these guidelines in Table 1.

For these ego-dystonic transgendered, the developmental history is different. Most patients remember episodes of cross-gendered expression or stated wishes early in their lives. They remember as well the swift disapproval that followed. If family and social sanctions had not been operative, they perhaps would have owned their cross-gendered identities sooner. Why this disapproval is effective in suppressing gender identity for the secondary group of patients and not for the primary group is not clear. It may be that the cross-gendered identity is not as strong or clear for the secondary group as it is for the primary transgendered. Nevertheless, these social role expectations become internalized, creating an ongoing state of internal conflict. The cross-gendered identity becomes ego-dystonic and the ego must rely on defense mechanisms such as suppression, repression, and dissociation to avoid fragmentation. As well, in order to gain social validation and reinforcement for the appropriate anatomic gender, participation in the stereotypically correct gender roles becomes of great importance. This includes heterosexual marriage (Table 2).

TABLE 1. Age Breakdown of Patients (271 Total)

	Age Range	Number	Percentage of Sample	Average Age (at first interview)
MTFP	15-60	58	21%	29.3
FTMP	16-34	22	8%	26.5
MTFS	21-61	162	60%	41
FTMS	21-52	29	11%	36.4

TABLE 2. Marriage History of Patients (271 Total)

	Number	Previously or Currently Married	Multiple Marriages
MTFP	58	0	
FTMP	22	0	
MTFS	162	105 (65%)	19 (12%)
FTMS	29	9 (31%)	0

For obvious reasons, the ego-syntonic transgendered do not marry conventionally before transition, as this would be participating in gender-appropriate role behavior. Since marriage gives social support against the unwanted internal identity, marriage for an MTFS or FTMS is an attempt to resolve conflict through a single action. Marriage provides as well an opportunity to have the company of a member of the gender one wishes to become. In other words, marriage provides an on-site same-sex friend with whom to identify. Many of these natal males are isolated in puberty and tend to marry the first compatible woman who accepts their proposal. If secret cross-dressing has been a means of decompressing their gender conflict, this may or may not be incorporated into the marriage. In clinical experience with patients seeking treatment for gender dysphoria, this attempt to resolve a gender conflict by marriage does not work. Most spouses want a marriage partner who assumes the complementary opposite sex roles, whereas most transgendered spouses are not very sexually active, and some marriages are almost celibate. Many patients report using dissociation in order to facilitate sexual intercourse. The transgendered assigned male becomes the woman who is receiving the penetration. The transgendered assigned female simply dissociates, removing herself from the situation into another place or perhaps viewing the intercourse from a distance. For the FTMS, marriage is less common than for the MTFS. These genetic women may adopt a lesbian identity for a while and form relationships in that context (Table 3).

Sexual orientation, based on gender identity, not anatomic or genetic identity, illustrates several variations. Three groups, the two primary groups and FTMS, identify themselves mostly as being heterosexual. For the primary transgendered, the percentage of homosexual orientation is only about 10%. In contrast, the MTFS group is more variable than the other three groups. The percentage of lesbianism is high. For many years these males have been striving to emulate the conventional male role as lover of females, and this appears to continue during and after their transitions. Eighteen percent state also that

TABLE 3. Sexual Orientation of Patients (271 Total) Based on Internal Gender Identity, Not Genetic or Anatomic Identity

	Number	Hetero	Homo	Bisexual	Does Not Know
MTFP	58	44 (76%)	7 (10%)	2 (3%)	5 (9%)
FTMP	20	20 (91%)	2 (9%)	0	0
MTFS	86	86 (53%)	46 (28%)	17 (10%)	13 (8%)
FTMS	21	21 (73%)	5 (17%)	1 (3%)	(7%)

they are bisexual or do not know what their preference is. Psychotherapy can help clear some of this confusion. However, for some in all four groups, sexual orientation will develop firmly only when they present totally in the gender they feel is authentic for them, meaning post-surgically, and receive the gender validation of sexual interest by others.

Because gender transition often includes periods of unclear or inconsistent gender presentation, it is a difficult time in respect to relationships. Erotic orientation being what it is, most people are attracted by definite gender signals. Gender ambiguity can be of interest to some, but it most usually causes avoidance. Must transgendered people transition without the support of a partner?

In Table 4, "an accepting partner" means someone of the erotically desired gender who knows and accepts the pre-surgical situation of the person in transition. As shown, about half of the members of three of the groups form these intimate relationships, and sometimes even manage to engineer legal marriages, e.g., an MTF marrying an FTM. In that situation, although the couple live in their desired cross-genders, they can marry legally if they are still legally natal male and female. The MTFS group is again the exception. They tend to go it alone. They reason that without the proper anatomy they cannot fully participate in the relationships they desire. This, however, does not hinder the other three groups from forming relationships. Isolation can be an issue for all transgendered patients but it is most common for the MTFS.

Further differences among the four groups appear in educational statistics (Table 5). Approximately one in ten of the MTFPs drop out of high school, either because of social pressures in school that become intolerable, or because they have run away from an intolerable situation in the home. This situation is avoidable as the following vignette demonstrates:

Asian-born D. was 17 when she was referred for evaluation by a local school board. Although D. was a good student, she could not stand the emotional and verbal abuse she suffered from her classmates in high school. Although assigned male, she consistently presented herself as female at school. With the support of her family and the school board, a plan was developed whereby D. would begin hormone therapy and reenter a different high school the next fall under a new female name. At follow up one year later, D. was extremely happy. She was graduating with honors and had dates to two different senior proms. Neither of her escorts knew she was not assigned female.

Support from D's family and the school system was crucial for this patient's well-being. Almost two-thirds of the MTFPs did not complete high school or stopped education at the high school level, compared to the more than half of the FTMPs who went on to college. Some of the MTFPs continue education later, as the following vignette illustrates, when they are more mature and more confident:

E., assigned male, had made her living preoperatively as a transsexual sex worker. At the age of 42, she began night courses at a local university as a female, and eight years later was awarded an associates degree with honors.

TABLE 4. Patients in a Primary Relationship with an Accepting Partner (271 Total)

	Total Number in Category	Number and Percentage
MTFP	58	23 (40%)
FTMP	22	30 (45%)
MTFS	162	43 (27%)
FTMS	29	13 (45%)

TABLE 5. Patients' Educational Level at First Interview (271 Total)

	Total	< High School	High School	College	Postgraduate
MTFP	58	5 (9%)	34 (58%)	18 (31%)	1 (< 1%)
FTMP	162	0	71 (44%)	74 (46%)	17 (10%)
MTFS	22	0	9 (41%)	12 (55%)	1 (4%)
FTMS	29	0	12 (41%)	11 (38%)	6 (21%)

The highest level of postgraduate education is in the secondary groups. Although this simply may be reflective of the older age of the population, for the MTFs it may also represent aggressive strivings to prove themselves within the male social role. An analogous motivation may exist for the FTMs who want to prove themselves highly competent in the other gender role.

Similar differences are seen when the occupational profile is examined (Table 6). The MTFPs have the highest lack of legitimate employment. Over one-third of them are self-admitted sex-workers or have no occupation. Of those with no occupation, some are indeed sex-workers, some are kept by male companions, and a few live at home. Obviously, they have a need for occupational and social assistance. By contrast, almost one-half of the FTMS group engage in professional level occupations. The older two groups in general have a higher level of employment, perhaps reflective of their age, their family responsibilities, and the use of hard aggressive work to try to suppress their unwanted cross-gender identities. Of interest are the two MTFS members of the armed forces who chose to begin transition while still in service. Both thought that joining the military would make men of them, in other words, make their female identification wither.

Joining the military, "workaholism," marriage with family, engaging in hypermasculine hobbies and sometimes dangerous pursuits are all common means by which the ego-dystonic transgendered person tries to control or even destroy the inner female identity:

> F., a thirty-eight-year-old female who is beginning her transition to male, not only bore two of her own children, but adopted three more. As she watched the party for her son's sixteenth birthday, she mused, "If I had done what I really had wanted to do all of my life, I would not be seeing this now."

Sometimes masculine hobbies are chosen because of side benefits:

> G., a MTFS, began to compete professionally in body-building in adolescence because "I could legitimately shave my body and get rid of that ugly hair!"

A problematic coping mechanism is the use of alcohol and other substances to quell the internal gender conflict (Table 7). The source of these figures is self-admission by the patients. The prevalence of drug/alcohol abuse in this population makes it imperative to obtain a history regarding substances. The two older secondary groups show prevalence approximately three times that of the national average. The link between substance abuse and GID in this

TABLE 6. Patients' Occupations (271 Total)

	MTFP (58)	FTMP (22)	MTFS (162)	FTMS (29)
None	13 (22%)	2 (9%)	21 (13%)	4 (14%)
Sex Worker	7 (12%)	0	3 (2%)	0
Student	7 (12%)	2 (9%)	5 (3%)	2 (7%)
Blue Collar	9 (15.5%)	6 (27%)	32 (20%)	1 (3.5%)
White Collar	12 (21%)	8 (36%)	44 (27%)	8 (28%)
Professional	7 (12%)	4 (18%)	50 (31%)	13 (45%)
Disabled	3 (5%)	0	3 (2%)	1 (3.5%)
Armed Forces	0	0	2 (1%)	0

TABLE 7. Positive History for Drug or Alcohol Abuse (271 Total)

	Number in Category	Number and Percentage
MTFP	58	18 (31%)
FTMP	22	3 (14%)
MTFS	162	57 (35%)
FTMS	29	9 (31%)

older population is the use of substances to suppress conflict. Some patients report that they became aware of their gender conflicts only after attaining sobriety. For others, the drug/alcohol usage became unnecessary once the previously unwanted gender identity became integrated into their personalities. The FTMP have not tried to suppress their internal male identity, did not need substances for that purpose, and thus have an incidence that resembles the national average. However, the other primary group, the MTFPs, do have a high incidence. Since they do not suppress their wishes to become female, their substance and alcohol abuse appears to originate in their lifestyle. Their use of drugs and alcohol appears clearly related to street life and prostitution.

Without question, drug and alcohol problems must be firmly under control before transition can be seriously considered:

When J. went for sexual reassignment surgery, her caregivers were unaware that she was still actively addicted to opiates. Two days post-surgically she went into major withdrawal and became unmanageable. She signed herself out of the hospital in order to seek drugs. The result of this was opening of unhealed tissues creating a recto-vaginal fistula. Reparative measures included a temporary colostomy, further prescribing of opiates, further drug-seeking, all of which created a spiral of surgery and opiates.

For the MTFs, primary and secondary, nicotine dependence also must be controlled because estrogen therapy increases the risk of deep vein thrombosis:

M., a 42-year-old Native American MTF, was a heavy smoker. Approximately six months after beginning estrogen therapy, she died suddenly while cleaning house. Evidently an embolus had originated in the deep veins in her legs.

The entire transgender population has a high usage rate of mental health services. Aside from the minimal therapy and counseling recommended in the *SOC*, many patients have had years of therapy in an attempt to deal with their internal struggle or their battles with society. This population is not immune to disorders that afflict the general population, but when the statistics here are examined, the transgender population shows a high incidence of concomitant disorders, mostly mood disorders. Unfortunately, the author's statistics have not yet been gathered to show the detailed breakdown of these other conditions. Without question, any co-existing disorder must be under control before transition is seriously underway. These secondary diagnoses are by history and/or evaluation on first visit (Table 8).

Some of the affective disorders lessen when the decision to transition is made, but this can also be only a temporary relief:

L., a 48-year-old MTF, told of a moment during her second marriage. "About eight years ago, I had my hunting rifle out. I was going to blow my head off or I was going to become a woman. Obviously I made the right decision. I haven't felt that depressed since."

SPECIFIC TREATMENT ISSUES

What are the specific treatment issues for each of these groups? MTFPs and FTMPs do not experience internal distress regarding their crossed identities. They are distressed regarding their unwanted primary and secondary sex char-

TABLE 8. Secondary Diagnoses Other Than Substance Abuse (271 Total)

	Number in Category	Number and Percentage
MTFP	58	23 (40%)
FTMP	22	7 (32%)
MTFS	162	61 (61%)
FTMS	29	10 (35%)

acteristics, but this distress is mitigated by the knowledge that anatomy can be changed. Their major source of distress is society's reaction to their strong cross-gendered expressions. Because they never suppress their internal identities, battles within the family regarding a child's rejection of appropriate roles start early and continue on. The FTMs seem to have fewer problems with their families, as it appears to be more acceptable to families to have a preadolescent tomboy than an effeminate son. However, the onset of puberty brings further struggles around clothing, brassieres, menses, and dating. These females often declare themselves to be lesbians as a means to cope with the family and social structure.

It is a different story for the MTFP. Feminine behavior in boys is poorly tolerated by all, and this intolerance of effeminacy sets the stage for emotional, physical, and sexual abuse. These young boys are labeled effeminate homosexuals early in life, producing further stigmatization. Unless the family can support a young transgendered male in his effort to express his female identity against social sanction, the only option for him might be to run away. The one advantage to this means of coping is that the young man might be able to contact others who can emphasize with him and understand him. Otherwise, this exposure to life on the street has little to offer:

L., a 44-year-old, came to the office to be evaluated for sexual reassignment surgery. She maintained that she had been born a "hermaphrodite" and at the age of six had had abdominal surgery to remove vestigial female organs. She had always felt that she basically was female and behaved in that manner. Her father felt that L. was an extreme embarrassment to him within the small community in which the family lived, and he beat L. frequently in an attempt to end such feminine behavior. At the age of sixteen, after a particularly brutal beating, L.'s mother gave her some money and a bus ticket and told her she must leave.

L. fled to the nearest large city, and there met other, older transgendered MTFs. They took L. in and trained her to be a transvestite entertainer, which became a highly successful career for her. Knowing that she must maintain her preoperative status to participate in her career, she had postponed genital surgery until she had saved enough money to change the direction of her life and pay for surgery. Simply by the strength of her personality, she had avoided the pitfalls of drugs, alcohol, and HIV.

The initial task for the therapist working with an ego-dystonic trans-gendered patient is to bring the split-off new identity to the foreground and facilitate integration into the personality. Some patients may need many years of therapy before they can comfortably start a transition. Beginning electrolysis and hormone therapy for males may provide a feeling that they are getting somewhere at last and therewith mitigate dysphoria in general. Because beginning testosterone for females produces changes that are difficult to reverse and cannot be hidden, such as deepening of the voice and facial/body hair, the FTMSs clearly must be ready to experience society's response to these changes. While these changes are welcome to FTMs, concurrent disorders must be under control. An individual who is struggling with a major disorder may not have the resilience to deal with this new situation.

After the ego-dystonic patient has integrated the new identity and dealt with internalized transphobia, he or she will have further complex situations to address. Although some general dysphoria and mild depression may lift when the decision to transition is made and initial results of hormone therapy are seen and felt, these patients usually are in for difficult times. Subsequent to beginning transition, there may be losses of family, children, and jobs. These losses are difficult to withstand, particularly for the individual who tends to respond to stress with depression:

> T., a 38-year-old FTM, was hospitalized for suicidal thinking before beginning transition. Her marriage of fifteen years had produced one child, a son, a 13-year-old at the time of hospitalization. During a family meeting with her wife, she blurted out that her problem was that she wanted to become a woman. "My wife stood up and said to me, 'Go ahead! You will never see your son again!' She walked out of the meeting. And I never saw my son again."

Since many of these people have dealt with their gender conflict by isolating, they may not have a wide network of support. For them, peer support as well as counseling is crucial. Thus, the older group, the ego-dystonic FTMs and MTFs, needs to revise more established and complex social situations that the younger group has not yet entered, such as marriage and established careers. But as a group, the older transgendered patients have more life experience, education, and resources with which to deal with potential loss and change. The high school dropout/runaway has few places to turn.

CONCLUSIONS

In summary, a patient population of 271 patients who meet the criteria for the diagnosis of GID has been divided into four relatively distinct groups. Natal assigned gender, male or female, creates the first division. The next division is based on whether or not the individual can suppress, or wants to suppress, an inner gender identity that conflicts with the assigned gender. Thus, within each group of male or female, are those for whom the inner identity is ego-syntonic and who tend to transition early, and those for whom the inner identity is ego-dystonic. These latter tend to transition later in life and perhaps could be considered as having GID, tardive type. By far, males transitioning to females are the most prevalent (81%, Table 1). The reason for this is not clear; it could be that it is more acceptable in this society for a woman to present a masculinized persona than it is for a man to present as feminine. For genetic women who may have GID, adopting a masculinized presentation may be sufficiently soothing to their gender dysphoria so that further action around the gender issue is not necessary, and therefore they do not seek treatment for GID. As stated above, the largest group is the secondary MTFs, perhaps in part reflective of the power social disapproval has in sanctioning feminine behavior in males, thus creating the conflict necessary to produce an ego-dystonic gender identity.

What all of these individuals share is that they meet the criteria for a *DSM-IV* diagnosis of GID. Before treatment, they live in a dissociated state of mind and body. The mind is of one gender, and the body is of the other. For most of them, neither the gender identity in the mind nor the anatomic sex of the body can be considered as pathologic. There is no recent clinical evidence that the gender identity can be changed through psychotherapy, even though the origin of gender identity is as yet unknown. However, the body can be changed, and when a proper transition to the other gender has been completed, the dissociation of GID disappears.

However, distinguishing these four groups has clinical significance in that each group has different therapeutic needs for specific interventions. Clearly, the younger patients, the MTFPs and FTMPs, need assistance with unaccepting and even estranged families. They often need help in dealing with educational systems that have difficulty integrating a student who shows gender deviant behavior. The MTFPs demonstrate the dangers resulting from dropping out of the family and schools. This group in particular is at high risk for disease and addiction. They frequently require vocational and educational help in order to develop a life off of the streets.

The older two groups, the MTFSs and FTMSs, initially need therapy to resolve the intrapsychic conflict regarding their internal identities so that they can reintegrate psychologically. Only then can transition truly begin. Subsequently, because many of them have created complex life situations that necessarily must change, they need the support of a therapeutic alliance to endure what can be extreme losses. If the patient has used isolation to cope with gender dysphoria, he or she may require assistance in developing basic social skills. Should these stresses activate an underlying disorder, medications will be of help.

Thus it seems, aside from validating the diagnosis and assisting in finding appropriate resources for transition, the main work of the therapist is helping the gender variant patient cope with the past and present psychological consequences of social stigma. The attempt to cure the basic problem ignites a chain reaction of severe social issues that can create enormous pain and suffering. Although the level of social acceptance has increased somewhat over the years, in most communities the transgendered minority has even fewer official protections than those afforded to gays and lesbians.

NOTE

1. The Harry Benjamin Association can be contacted at HIBIGDA@FRAMPRAC. UMN.edu.

REFERENCES

American Psychiatric Association (1987), *Diagnostic and Statistical Manual of Mental Disorders, Third Edition, Revised.* Washington, DC: American Psychiatric Association.

_____ (1994), *Diagnostic and Statistical Manual of Psychiatric Disorders, Fourth Edition.* Washington, DC: American Psychiatric Association.

Bakker, A., von Kesteren, P.J.M., Gooren, L.J.G. & Bezemer, P.D. (1993), The prevalence of transsexualism in the Netherlands. *Acta Psychiatr. Scand.*, 87:237-238.

Meyer W., Bockting, W., Cohen-Kettenis, P., Coleman, E., DiCeglie, D., Devor, H., Gooren, L., Hage, J., Kirk, S., Kuiper, B., Laub, D., Lawrence, A., Menard, Y., Patton, J., Schaefer, L., Webb, A. & Wheeler, C. (2001), The standards of care for gender identity disorders, sixth version. *Int. J. Transgenderism* 5(1):http//www. symposion.com/ijt/soc_1

Guilt in Cross Gender Identity Conditions: Presentations and Treatment

Leah Cahan Schaefer, EdD
Connie Christine Wheeler, PhD

SUMMARY. Guilt in cross gender conditions is one of the most difficult manifestations of inner conflict to identify and measure accurately. While developing psychometric measurements of guilt in gender identity conditions in adults, the authors noted recurring themes in virtually all clients in their clinical practice over the past 25 years. To test their initial impressions of themes of guilt, the authors gathered data from both clinical experience and from research studies specifically designed to identify areas in which patients reported feelings of guilt. Data were gathered on a total of 787 patients, of which 685 were pre- and 102 post-operative. They found 13 themes of guilt in their subjects. The authors believe that understanding the primary sources of the special kind

Leah Cahan Schaefer is a psychologist in private practice in New York City. She has specialized in the treatment of gender dysphoria conditions since 1975.

Connie Christine Wheeler, a psychologist specializing in Human Sexuality, is in private practice in New York City.

Both Dr. Schaefer and Dr. Wheeler were charter members of the Harry Benjamin International Gender Dysphoria Association. Dr. Schaefer served as President of the organization for two terms. Dr. Wheeler has served as HBIGDA's Secretary-Treasurer, and currently sits on the Board of Directors.

Address correspondence to: Leah C. Schaefer, EdD, 285 Riverside Drive, New York, NY 10025 or Connie Christine Wheeler, PhD, New York University, 310 East 46 Street, Suite 12-H, New York, NY 10017 (E-mail: christinewheeler@msn.com).

[Haworth co-indexing entry note]: "Guilt in Cross Gender Identity Conditions: Presentations and Treatment." Schaefer, Leah Cahan, and Connie Christine Wheeler. Co-published simultaneously in *Journal of Gay & Lesbian Psychotherapy* (The Haworth Medical Press, an imprint of The Haworth Press, Inc.) Vol. 8, No. 1/2, 2004, pp. 117-127; and: *Transgender Subjectivities: A Clinician's Guide* (ed: Ubaldo Leli, and Jack Drescher) The Haworth Medical Press, an imprint of The Haworth Press, Inc., 2004, pp. 117-127. Single or multiple copies of this article are available for a fee from The Haworth Document Delivery Service [1-800-HAWORTH, 9:00 a.m. - 5:00 p.m. (EST). E-mail address: docdelivery@haworthpress.com].

Digital Object Identifer: 10.1300/J236v08n01_09

of guilt connected with gender dysphoria is crucial to understanding the gender dysphoric person. A major goal of their treatment is the elimination of the crippling effects of guilt. One of the authors offers examples from her clinical practice for this approach to psychotherapy. *[Article copies available for a fee from The Haworth Document Delivery Service: 1-800-HAWORTH. E-mail address: <docdelivery@haworthpress.com> Website: <http://www.HaworthPress.com> © 2004 by The Haworth Press, Inc. All rights reserved.]*

KEYWORDS. Gender dysphoria, gender identity disorder, guilt, psychometric measures, psychotherapy, sex reassignment, transgender, transsexual

INTRODUCTION

Although guilt is an ancient topic of philosophical inquiry and certainly not new to analytic examination, few papers make reference to its importance in gender identity conditions (Guze, 1969; Wheeler and Schaefer, 1984; Schaefer, Wheeler, and Futterweit, 1995). Despite the paucity of allusions to gender dysphoric guilt in the literature, guilt is often the motivating factor that dictates how gender-distressed persons interpret, manage, and live their lives. The definition of guilt, how to recognize it, how to measure it, and how to gauge its impact on identity are central issues that cannot be overemphasized in both the diagnosis and the treatment of gender dysphoria.

Gender conditions (transsexualism, transgenderism, transvestism, gender dysphoria, gender identity disorders) represent a person's desire to live, to be known, and to be accepted as a member of a sex different from the one assigned at birth. They are usually accompanied by a sense of discomfort with one's anatomic sex and a wish to have hormonal treatment and surgery to make one's body as congruent as possible with the preferred sex (Benjamin, 1966).

Guilt is the state of one who has committed an offense. It motivates morbid self-reproach, and often manifests in marked preoccupation with the moral correctness of one's behavior. Guilt may leave a person feeling unfit even to exist. A person who feels guilty feels subversive, larcenous, and justly liable to burden, forfeiture, and remorse. What is the origin of guilt in the cross gender identity phenomenon? The authors believe that the origin of such guilt stems from each gender non-conforming person's lack of understanding of the source of his or her dilemma, and the implied self-blame.

In the context of this paper, the reference to people as "patients" is used to identify both the established medical nature of Gender Identity Disorder

(GID), and the relationship of those seeking consultation to the various treatments and services received from physicians, psychologists, and other health care practitioners. The language is not intended to pathologize.

Guilt surfaces in gender disordered children, usually between the ages of 3 and 9, as they become aware that they are not like other boys or other girls. Children fear being "different" because difference can lead to rejection by family, friends, and other social groups. They conclude that there is something wrong with them. With this realization, a sense of secretiveness takes over, characterized by the twin preoccupations, "Nobody must know," and "Am I giving myself away?" Shame follows, because such a secret is not one to be proud of, or to share with others. With shame comes blame. Whose fault is this? If something is wrong, there must be a culprit; someone must be blamed. Since the emotion emanates internally, the child can blame no one but itself: "It must be me. I must have done something bad, or wrong, or sinful to be so different from others." The emotional focus is on wrong, and subsequently on punishment. This pattern, consistently demonstrated in our practices, irrevocably solidifies guilt, a guilt that necessitates recompense.

It is essential to remember that this type of guilt derives from no *act* committed, but from simply the way one is. It seems appropriate therefore, to call this an existential guilt, resulting from an existential crime, the self-perceived crime of existence, which leads to a lifetime of defensive habits set up to "pay" for the sin of existing. Restitution is experienced in patterns of isolation, victimization, feelings of profound worthlessness and shame, a sense of not belonging, and a chronic need to apologize for oneself. Gender dysphoric persons learn to deny that they even have a self, other than guilt personified, which creates in them the feeling of being both victim and executioner. Such feelings inhibit progressive emotional and personal identity growth. The sources of this guilt and its ramifications are difficult to identify even by the adult gender dysphoric person.

Guilt, in cross gender conditions, is one of the most difficult manifestations of inner conflict to identify and measure accurately. While developing psychometric measurements of guilt in gender identity conditions in adults, the authors noted recurring themes in virtually all clients in their clinical practice over the past 25 years. To test their initial impressions of themes of guilt, the authors gathered data from both clinical experience and from research studies specifically designed to identify areas in which patients reported feelings of guilt. Two ongoing research studies were initiated to explore and define guilt and its descriptors in gender dysphoric conditions. Key questions in the research studies–later explored in clinical work with patients–asked what forms guilt took in relation to gender feelings on a daily basis, and at the time when the patients initially recognized being gender variant.

METHODOLOGY AND SAMPLE

An item pool of guilt in cross gender identity conditions was constructed from descriptions of guilt collected in clinical interviews, and from the written descriptions of research participants in the two ongoing studies. Data were gathered on a total of 787 patients, of which 685 were pre- and 102 post-operative. Reports by clinical research participants were consistent with those of clients in clinical practice.

The authors and two anonymous knowledgeable researchers on guilt, who served as blind independent raters, carried out initial content analysis. Thematic segments were identified, yielding a breakdown to 13 categories of guilt content, with corresponding definitions. A jury of three additional experts reviewed the categories and definitions, and unanimously agreed that the categories, titles, and definitions were appropriate to the guilt themes.

RESULTS

Although it is not the purpose of this paper to report fully on these two studies in progress, preliminary findings reconfirm the usefulness of psychotherapeutic treatment of guilt in gender dysphoria.

Exploration of the forms that guilt takes identifies thirteen major types described in Table 1. Although these thirteen categories include the most prominent descriptors of guilt for virtually all individuals with whom the authors have worked over the past twenty-seven years, they should not be considered all inclusive. Some overlap between types of guilt expressed was observed. The sheer number of gender dysphoric people (1,387 in the authors' clinical practices) and the frequency with which the authors have heard similar expressions of guilt supports the clinical usefulness of these categories. Their variety and scope illustrate how pervasive guilt is in the life of the gender dysphoric person, encompassing all areas of human relationships and interactions.

Among transsexual patients who had undergone genital restructuring surgery, there was a significant amount of residual guilt, which these individuals carried with themselves despite their frequently reported belief that surgery would have solved all their problems. All 102 clients studied had surgery before the advent of the *Standards of Care (SOC)* (Schaefer and Wheeler, 1995; Meyer et al., 2001), which requires psychotherapy with a health care provider with special training in the area of gender identity disorders before undertaking the process of transition. All the post-operative individuals still suffered from unresolved guilt, which resulted in an emotional paralysis that made them feel misunderstood and fearful of opening up to social and/or sexual relationships.

TABLE 1. Categories of Guilt in Cross-Gender Conditions (From Most to Least Frequently Expressed)

1) NOT BEING NORMAL	Not feeling that one fits into the standard image of a male or female, thus deviating from acceptable norms.
2) WHAT OTHERS MIGHT THINK	Projected fear of non-acceptance of one's condition onto others. Fear of "being read" or being found out.
3) APPEARING TO BE ONE GENDER, BUT FEELING ANOTHER	Sense of deceiving others by not revealing one's gender condition, gender history, or one's preferred inner gender self. Guilt in prior real life experience, as well as prolonged life experience, often heightened by fear of discovery or disclosure.
4) DISAPPOINTMENT CAUSED TO FAMILY OR EXTENDED FAMILY (including therapists, physicians, and other health care providers)	Sense of failure to fulfill others' realizations, hopes and desires.
5) DEPRIVING OTHERS	By not fulfilling the expected, "acceptable" role(s), one assumes responsibility for hurting others by wanting, or needing, to be oneself.
6) ASSUMPTION OF CRITICISM	Sense of being wrong, blameworthy, and deserving of attack, and thus ultimately never accepted by others.
7) BLAME FOR SOMETHING NOT ONE'S FAULT	Assumption of responsibility for complaints and accusations by others, regardless of actual culpability. One makes excuses.
8) NEED FOR APPROVAL	Desire for authoritative sanction, confirmation, and/or validation, in order to relieve guilt.
9) SELF-DEPRIVATION	Sense of unworthiness of acceptance, happiness, or peace of mind.
10) SEXUAL FEELINGS	Guilt regarding erotic thoughts and their expression. Although other clinical populations may be similarly erotophobic, homophobic, and/or gender-phobic, transgendered patients often mistake these feelings as deriving from their gender condition.
11) RELIGIOUS OR SPIRITUAL	One feels bound by quasi-monastic vows, dictates, or rules, and senses a necessity to fulfill absolute obligations to the teachings of whatever religious faith, or spiritual belief, one adheres to.
12) NOT FEELING GUILT	In a state of denial, one is unable to recognize resistance to acknowledging guilt, although some may agree to feeling shame.
13) PERPETUAL PAYMENT	One assuages guilt by a lifetime of constant restitution. Continual suffering or anxiety is fundamental in all forms of payment.

These persons never had the benefit of a special psychotherapy that could have helped them to be aware of the impact of guilt in all areas of their lives. They believed that simply having the sex reassignment surgery would resolve all the difficulties that they had experienced throughout their lives. They seemed unable to understand that the genital re-sculpting surgery would only resolve one major area of difficulty by establishing an accord between their inner understanding of their gender and their appearance.

One 67-year-old woman (25 years post-op) has still not had highly desired, longed-for sexual intercourse with a male for fear of still being discovered or recognized as a transsexual–this, despite the fact that upon each of her employer's mandatory biannual physical examinations the condition of her internal genitalia has been reported by the physicians as post-hysterectomy.

A very beautiful and successful 40-year-old transsexual woman (2 years post-op) came to therapy wanting to learn how to attract a man. She admitted to feeling shame, but not guilt. She said, "I don't believe that guilt would cause me to advertise my condition any more than being an ax murderer, for example, would lead one to have that information branded across one's forehead." The therapist expressed amazement that this person found being a transsexual comparable to being an ax murderer. She sat back laughing and said, "Touché!"

Another person likened her situation to being a part of the FBI Witness Protection Program, wherein identifying characteristics are gradually stripped away to create a new persona for protection from the world. One 54-year-old (25 years post-op) FTM transsexual in the middle of a great depression wrote 13 pages of "What's wrong with me" and "What a terrible person I am," only to realize that his self-recrimination was based on feelings of sinfulness and guilt, and not on actions.

Finally, one very eloquent patient (age 54, who lives as the non-natal gender, although without having had surgery) stated:

> I have found both relief and satisfaction in reclaiming myself. However, the process is one I live and work at everyday–in fact, the process is my life itself. But the guilt feelings go so deep it's hard to hold on to my self-esteem and myself. I finally learned about making relationships, and feel I've aligned myself with really good things. Yet it seems so easy to fall into traps, settle and give up on positive things. At this moment, in terms of the human condition, my life sucks and is not working. By all appearances, I seemingly have everything–everything except me!

The intense influence of guilt and its accompanying feelings of anxiety is so powerful that it affects even the feelings of many of the significant others who live, play, or work with gender dysphoric people. The issue of gender–so utterly fundamental to the development and understanding of the human personality–is one which arouses incredible anxiety in most people asked to understand or tolerate any variations in the concept of what is male or female: they find it confusing to place people with a gender dysphoria condition.

The families of the gender dysphoric person are especially affected by guilt. There are families that often would prefer that their dysphoric child be homosexual, in order to avoid the extreme changes–hormones and sex reassignment surgery–which make the condition more visible to others. There are parents who are relieved to learn about the possibility of prenatal influence on gender conditions, so that they need not feel guilty for their child's rare and misunderstood dilemma.

These families do not understand the accidental, but natural, cause of this phenomenon, tend to perceive it as a sexual (genital related) anomaly, and therefore find it confusing and embarrassing. They feel that they themselves have suffered and have had to tolerate so much, just from having the gender dysphoric person in their midst, that they often become intolerant and unsupportive of their gender distressed relative. The patients feel rejected and misunderstood, and seek someone else from whom to receive empathy and acceptance. Often this person is their therapist.

Guilt affects still other significant people in the lives of the gender-dysphoric. The authors interviewed some active practitioners in the field of cross gender identity disorders about feelings of guilt regarding their patients' conditions. Very few professionals understood well the subtleties of the conditions' manifestations–that they are not conditions of choice; that they continue for the patients' lifetimes; and that there are many options and alternatives for treatment. Some even believed that if a patient were not likely to present an attractive appearance, all effort made to live in the preferred gender role would be useless, might negate the diagnosis, and, ultimately, disqualify the potential candidate for hormones or surgery.

TREATMENT IMPLICATIONS

The *SOC* require, among other interventions, that each person spend one to two years in psychotherapy in order to prepare for transitioning to their preferred gender role, including obtaining sex reassignment surgery (Levine, 1999). The mental health care provider's role is of fundamental importance because, of all the professionals providing services, it is the therapist who will spend the longest time working with the gender dysphoric person. Consequently, it is the psychotherapist who will have the most influence on their education, guidance, understanding, progress, and development.

The content of the psychotherapy required is not spelled out specifically in the *SOC*, but whatever form the treatment takes should include a consideration of the crucial impact that guilt has on gender dysphoria. Gender variance will emerge with varying intensity throughout one's life, independently of attempts to suppress or deny it. Psychotherapy cannot eradicate it. There is no choice about who one wants to be; the only choice is how one wants to live.

The authors believe that understanding the primary sources of the special kind of guilt connected with gender dysphoria is crucial to understanding the gender dysphoric person. We believe the guilt develops between the ages of 2 or 3, when the child first learns words to express its inner feelings; and at age 10 or 11, when secondary sex characteristics become visible. With education through therapy, the gender dysphoric person can understand that her/his gender condition is an accidental, but valid birth phenomenon. Without this understanding, it is likely that the gender dysphoric person will feel blameworthy, or, as one person describes it, "guilt personified." Feelings of guilt originate out of ignorance, but the guilt eventually vanishes with understanding.

Cross gender identified people frequently do not recognize the all-pervasive contamination that feelings of guilt have caused at every level of their lives. A major goal of our treatment is the elimination of the crippling effects of guilt. The techniques we employ in the psychotherapy process specifically focusing on guilt include teaching by example, by experience, by role-playing, by reflecting, by identification; joining with others in support groups; and constant, exploration, reevaluation, validation, and confirmation.

One of the authors (LCS), who has worked with gender dysphoric people for more than 25 years, has devised a holistic system of educational psychotherapy aimed at lessening or eliminating the guilt phenomenon, which addresses the psychological needs of gender dysphoric people whose growth has been impeded by the special guilt with which they have been burdened. The therapy is primarily designed to educate, or rather, re-educate the patient by studying the Story of His/Her Life. Most often, it is quite a different story than one has been aware of–a story which begins with the first awareness (usually between the ages of 3 and 9) that one is not like other boys or other girls. The same author (LCS) believes, in fact, that the story begins even earlier than this first awareness. It begins in the first moments after birth, when the delivering doctor (or other birth assistant) first identifies the gender of the new baby according to the appearance of the genitalia. With a gender dysphoric person, this is truly a case of mistaken identity. As a result of this unintended error, the child will hence be forced to live in a gender that feels completely uncomfortable and unsuitable. Note that it is confusion, mistakes, and misunderstandings that cause gender dysphoric people to develop the guilt with which they become saddled from childhood on. Because they recognize that they are not like other boys or other girls, they feel–universally, in LCS's experience–that something is *wrong* with them, and that it must be the result of something wrong they have done. There is no one to blame–not God, not even their mother, only themselves. Thus begins the guilt. The fact that the experience of gender dysphoria, at least in childhood, is usually kept a secret perhaps explains why guilt is also internally focused. The guilt caused by these early experiences, however, is not the only guilt that gender dysphoric people experience. Because they have an overwhelming need to find a way to their true gender, they begin, for instance, to cross-dress. This behavior, while satisfying to them, is so outside the norms of our society that it creates more anxiety and more guilt.

The therapist can help the patient understand his or her story, and also to realize that no one–least of all the patient–is at fault for this accident of birth. Through the course of the therapy, the patient will arrive at sessions with many different presenting issues. These issues may be directly related to the gender condition, or they may be related to some other aspect of daily or emotional life. At the core of nearly all the difficulties gender dysphoric people experience, however, is guilt. The therapist's task is to expose the guilt that underlies whatever may be troubling the patient, or causing problems in the ability to function successfully, and then to help the patient connect the feelings of guilt associated with a particular problem to the primary guilt feelings, which are gender-related. The therapist repeatedly aids the patient in reconnecting primary and secondary guilt feelings, until a new understanding has been integrated. This can happen only in an atmosphere of acceptance, in which the patient and therapist are able to form a therapeutic alliance. In such an atmosphere, the therapist can encourage the patient to feel more comfortable in, for instance, cross-dressing, and ultimately less guilty about such behavior. The patient can then enjoy the satisfaction and peace that cross-dressing often provides.

Gender dysphoric people often are not accustomed to feeling acceptance and understanding from others–bosses, family members, etc.–and therefore tend at first not to trust such acceptance, even when coming from a therapist. Patients are often not aware that they themselves tend to reject or push away friendly, affirmation overtures. It is useful for the therapist to make the patient aware of this tendency, and to help him or her to accept positive feelings from the therapist, and eventually from others. One patient, when asked, toward the end of treatment, what it was that had made the work together so successful, responded:

> At first I had a very hard time believing that what you were telling were the real facts, and not what I had believed for so long. But eventually, when I did, my whole life eased up and everything got better and more manageable and acceptable. Also, the very way that you accepted me and my efforts–how you encouraged me to come to a session "dressed"– it was the first time I went out that way– and how you complimented me

on my outfit and my makeup, my hair and everything. I felt that you gave me a new lease on life–which also encouraged my wife to be more accepting, too!

A note of caution in treating guilt in the gender dysphoric person. Guilt cannot be treated as separate from all other issues related to the gender conditions. The earliest concept of self a transgender person has is one of a totally guilt-ridden image–a "self with no self." A therapist cannot treat a gender dysphoric person by separating the patient's problems from the earliest perception of how they developed, with the accompanying feelings of torment, isolation, shame, and, for those who are religious, of being forgotten or overlooked by God. Once the cross-gender identity-guilt condition is understood and accepted, one can say, as did the psychoanalyst at the conclusion of Philip Roth's Portnoy's Complaint, "Now we can begin" (p. 274).

CONCLUSIONS

Gender identity conditions are filled with myths and misinformation and misconceptions. The major answer to the ultimate understanding and acceptance of these rare conditions is education. Only through education can prejudices be lifted and truths emerge. Our colleague and friend, Harry Benjamin, M.D., wrote, "Instead of treating the patient, might it not be wiser and more sensible to treat society educationally, so that logic, understanding, and compassion might prevail?" (Benjamin, 1953)

The authors have long felt that androgynous perceptions–that aspect in all of us, which includes some maleness and some femaleness–may indeed be the highest form of true gender development. As other researchers have noted, gender blending is a satisfying way of life for some people (Devor, 1989). One of the obstacles that prevents most transgender people from achieving their own highest levels of development is the interference in their growth caused by pervasive and pernicious guilt, the influence of which we have tried here to describe. Our experience with gender dysphoric patients demonstrates that the elimination of the influence of guilt allows for a more satisfying and more productive life for members of this remarkable population.

REFERENCES

Benjamin, H. (1953), Transvestism in the news. *J. Am. Med. Assoc.*, 1:56.
_____ (1966), *The Transsexual Phenomenon*. New York, NY: Julian Press.
Devor, H. (1989), *Gender Blending: Confronting the Limits of Duality*. Bloomington and Indianapolis, IN: Indiana University Press.

Guze, H. (1969), Psychosocial adjustment of transsexuals: An evaluation and theoretical formulation. In: *Transsexualism and Sex Reassignment*, eds. R. Green & J. Money. Baltimore, MD: Johns Hopkins Press, pp. 171-181.

Levine, S.B. (1999), The newly revised STANDARDS OF CARE for gender identity disorders. *J. Sex Educ. & Ther.*, 24:117-127.

Meyer W., Bockting, W., Cohen-Kettenis, P., Coleman, E., DiCeglie, D., Devor, H., Gooren, L., Hage, J., Kirk, S., Kuiper, B., Laub, D., Lawrence, A., Menard, Y., Patton, J., Schaefer, L., Webb, A. & Wheeler, C. (2001), *Standards of Care for Gender Identity Disorders, Sixth version*. Düsseldorf, Germany: Symposium Publications.

Roth, P. (1994), *Portnoy's Complaint*. New York: Vintage.

Schaefer, L.C. & Wheeler, C.C. (1995), Clinical historical notes: Harry Benjamin's first ten cases (1938-1953). *Arch. Sex. Behav.*, 24:73-93.

———, ——— & Futterweit, W. (1995), Gender identity disorders (transsexualism). In: *Treatments Of Psychiatric Disorders, Second Edition*, ed. G. Gabbard. Washington, DC: American Psychiatric Press, pp. 2015-2079.

Wheeler, C.C. & Schaefer, L.C. (1984), The nonsurgery true transsexual (Benjamin's category IV): A theoretical rationale. In: *International Research In Sexology: Sexual Medicine, Vol. 1 (Selected Papers from the Fifth World Congress of Sexology)*, eds. H. Lief & Z. Hoch. New York, NY: Praeger, pp. 167-174.

Disclosure, Risks and Protective Factors for Children Whose Parents Are Undergoing a Gender Transition

Tonya White, MD
Randi Ettner, PhD

SUMMARY. *Objective:* This study attempts to delineate the effects on children within different stages of development whose parent undergoes a transition to the other sex.

Methods: Questionnaires were mailed to therapists who have considerable experience working with gender dysphoric patients. These therapists were queried about their experience with individuals who had children prior to the start of their transition. Variables such as the nature and manner of disclosure to the child and the nature of the relationships between the child and each parent were evaluated.

Results: Children in the preschool years were rated as adapting best to

Tonya White is Assistant Professor, Division of Child and Adolescent Psychiatry, University of Minnesota, and Research Consultant, New Health Foundation. Her research interests include the use of neuroimaging tools to study functional brain connectivity in normal development and in pediatric neuropsychiatric disorders.

Randi Ettner is President of New Health Foundation, an organization founded to assist the transgendered. She is a member of the American Psychological Association, the American College of Forensic Psychologists, the University of Chicago Gender Board, and the Harry Benjamin Gender Dysphoria Association.

Address correspondence to: Randi Ettner, PhD, New Health Foundation, 1214 Lake Street, Evanston, IL 60201 (E-mail: rettner@aol.com).

[Haworth co-indexing entry note]: "Disclosure, Risks and Protective Factors for Children Whose Parents Are Undergoing a Gender Transition." White, Tonya, and Randi Ettner. Co-published simultaneously in *Journal of Gay & Lesbian Psychotherapy* (The Haworth Medical Press, an imprint of The Haworth Press, Inc.) Vol. 8, No. 1/2, 2004, pp. 129-145; and: *Transgender Subjectivities: A Clinician's Guide* (ed: Ubaldo Leli, and Jack Drescher) The Haworth Medical Press, an imprint of The Haworth Press, Inc., 2004, pp. 129-145. Single or multiple copies of this article are available for a fee from The Haworth Document Delivery Service [1-800-HAWORTH, 9:00 a.m. - 5:00 p.m. (EST). E-mail address: docdelivery@haworthpress.com].

the transition, both initially and long-term. Adults also were able to adapt well, so long as the level of conflict between parents was low. Adolescents had the most difficult time adapting to a parental transition. The level of family conflict worsened the child's adaptation across all developmental levels. The therapists delineated both risk and protective factors for children during such a situation.

Conclusions: While a parent undergoing a gender transition is not a neutral event, both risk and protective factors do exist, and knowledge of these may be beneficial in assisting the child's adaptation to the situation. Adolescents appear to have the most difficult time adapting to a parental transition and extra support may be needed for this group. These findings are discussed in light of identified resilience factors in children and approaches that therapists can employ to best assist families found in such a situation. Case examples are provided. *[Article copies available for a fee from The Haworth Document Delivery Service: 1-800-HAWORTH. E-mail address: <docdelivery@haworthpress.com> Website: <http://www. HaworthPress.com>* © *2004 by The Haworth Press, Inc. All rights reserved.]*

KEYWORDS. Adolescent, child, divorce, gender dysphoria, gender identity disorder, gender role, gender transition, GID, parenting, sexual reassignment, transgender, transsexual

INTRODUCTION

Although individuals with gender dysphoria have been present since antiquity, the medical advances within the past seventy years have dramatically expanded both the understanding and the potential treatments for these conditions. Residing on the far end of the spectrum of gender dysphoria is a condition known as Gender Identity Disorder (GID). The *Diagnostic and Statistical Manual, Fourth Edition (DSM-IV)* defines GID in adolescents and adults as a persistent desire to live as a member of the other sex (American Psychiatric Association, 1994, pp. 532-538). This preoccupation is manifest by an intense desire to adopt the social role and to acquire the physical appearance of the other sex. These individuals are uncomfortable being regarded by others as, or functioning in society as a member of their designated sex and thus often seek hormonal and surgical treatments to alleviate their discordance.

GID is a relatively uncommon condition with an approximate incidence between 1 in 11,900 to 45,000 in males and 1 in 30,000 to 100,000 in females (American Psychiatric Association, 1994, pp. 532-538; van-Kesteren, Gooren and Megens, 1996; Weitze and Osburg, 1996). Between 43% to 50% of transsexual patients will choose nonsurgical solutions (Green and Blanchard, 2000;

Keller, Althof, and Lothstein, 1982). Approximately 77-80% of diagnosed transsexuals who present to a gender identity clinic will ultimately undergo hormonal therapy and/or sexual reassignment surgery (van-Kesteren, Gooren, and Megens, 1996). Of those who do progress through surgery, outcome studies of GID have demonstrated that such intervention can alleviate the gender dysphoria and emotional comorbidity in 68% to 97% of the individuals (Fahrner, Kockott, and Duncan, 1987; Pauly, 1981; Rakic et al., 1996; Tsoi, 1993).

Of the genetic males who enter treatment, approximately 50% are either married or have been married, and approximately 70% of these have had children. Genetic females with GID are typically less likely to enter marriages with males and are also less likely to have borne children. Nevertheless, it does occur, and in both scenarios children are placed in an atypical situation within the present cultural milieu. There is a paucity of research describing the effects of a parental gender transposition on children and adolescents.

In a study of 37 children of either transsexual or homosexual parents, Green (1978) reported that these children did not differ appreciably from those raised in more conventional family settings. Of the 16 children in homes with transsexuals, 7 were raised with male-to-female transsexuals and 9 were raised with female-to-male transsexuals. The age range of the children in the homes of transsexuals was 3 to 20 years (mean 11.3) and the duration that they had lived in the home ranged from 1 to 16 years (mean 6.76). In most cases, the children were aware of the parent's gender transition and the majority had witnessed the transition. Green's work focused on issues of gender identity, role, and sexuality rather than overall development and issues of adaptation, family, school, and peer interactions. Furthermore, a control group was not included in the study. Green (1998b) had a second study on the topic with similar findings. A recent case report described the successful intervention in a child whose father was undergoing a transition from the male to the female gender role (Sales, 1995). A thorough review of the literature failed to elicit any further research on this topic. Thus, the summary of the effects on children whose parent undertakes a gender transposition can be summarized in one paragraph.

Children are born into families with a gender dysphoric parent for a myriad of reasons. Common reasons include an attempt by the parent to live according to the assigned gender role due to social pressure or in hope that the dysphoria will somehow resolve over time. There is no evidence that this acceptance of the assigned gender role alters an individual's core gender identity and an unknown percentage will pursue a gender role transition. A small fraction of these families, mainly with male-to-female transsexuals, will remain as an intact family throughout such a transition. Equating children from families who remain intact with those who do not would be unwise, as families who work together in this area may well be more apt to present a unified explanation of the transition to the children. In fact, families who remain intact are likely to have more similarities to homosexual families than to families who separate or divorce.

A number of studies have evaluated the effects of children raised within homosexual families. Reports reveal both negative (Crawford and Solliday, 1996) and neutral attitudes (Maney and Cain, 1997). Males and those with stronger religious attitudes had more negative attitudes toward homosexual families (Maney and Cain, 1997). Although a bias exists against awarding custody to homosexual parents (Allen and Burrell, 1996; Brewaeys and van-Hall, 1997; Kleber, Howell, and Tibbits-Kleber, 1986; van-Nijnatten, 1995), nearly all studies reported that children raised in homosexual families are no different in psychological, social, or sexual development (Allen and Burrell, 1996; Brewaeys and van-Hall, 1997; Gold, Perrin, and Futterman, 1994; Green, 1986; Patterson, 1992; Tasker and Golombok, 1995). One study that combined single-female-headed and lesbian households found that the children within these homes experienced greater warmth and interaction with their mother and were more securely attached to her. However, they perceived themselves as less cognitively and physically competent than those families with a father present (Golombok, Tasker, and Murray, 1997).

In many, but not all, marriages in which a spouse enters a transition to the other sex, the process results in eventual divorce. With considerable information describing the effects of divorce on children, it becomes somewhat difficult to tease apart the adverse consequences of separation and divorce as separate from the gender transition itself. This is further complicated by studies that reveal that the impact of a highly conflicted divorce in the context of violent relationships can precipitate separation and individuation difficulties, as well as disturbances of gender and sexual identity in children (Wallerstein and Corbin, 1996). A number of transsexuals who initiated families during their earlier years in attempts at normalcy will choose to await the growth of their children to adulthood prior to initiating their transition. Understanding that children may actually fare better when parental separation or divorce spares them from further domestic hostility, the picture becomes less clear when the life of a child is complicated by a parent with untreated gender dysphoria. There have been no studies to date addressing the latter.

Males and females react differently to divorce (Hetherington, Cox, and Cox, 1982; Wallerstein and Kelly, 1980; Zaslow, 1988, 1989). Whereas typical sex-role typing in girls did not appear to be disrupted by divorce, boys scored lower on male preference and higher on female preference on testing of sex-role determinants (Wallerstein and Corbin, 1996). Boys also tended to spend more time playing with girls and younger children and tested significantly below a matched control group from intact families in academic achievement and social relationships (Wallerstein and Corbin, 1996). The role of the custodial parent may prove important in this regard, as school age children demonstrated greater sociability and independence when custody was granted to the same sex parent in comparison with those children in which the opposite sex parent was the custodial parent (Santrock and Warshak, 1979).

There is evidence of increased need for the father by both adolescent boys and girls and that feelings of rejection at this period of development may pose difficulties for the teenager (Wallerstein and Corbin, 1996). Girls have reported to have more difficulties during the adolescent and early adult years with notable difficulties in separating from their mothers (Kalter, Reimer, and Brickman, 1985; Wallerstein and Blakeslee, 1989). It is unclear to date the psychological and developmental effects on children when a gender transition of the parent is coupled with divorce. Given the complications of a hostile divorce, it is likely that a gender transition in the context of an intact family bears little consequence when compared to non-gender dysphoric parents in the midst of a conflicted divorce. However, coupling of a conflicted divorce scenario with a parent undergoing a gender transition may well amplify the children's difficulties (see case study of Manuel). This may be especially noteworthy in the context of a hostile parental relationship and children who are the same genetic sex of the transitioning parent.

When parents alter their relationship in such a manner that the children's contact with either parent is reduced, either by separation or divorce, specific protective and risk factors have been determined (American Academy of Pediatrics, 1996). Children who appear to be more at risk include those who: (i) have a close emotional relationship with the noncustodial parent; (ii) experience childhood guilt about believing one is the cause of the marital discord; (iii) experience a sudden and unexplained divorce; (iv) endures greater hostility in relationships; (v) experience persistent conflict and litigation (particularly about custody); and (vi) have a parent with a mental illness. Children who fare better with parental separation or divorce tend to have a number of protective factors which include: (i) consistent explanation and exoneration of the child; (ii) absence of litigation and parental discord; (iii) ongoing contact with both parents; (iv) sparing children from the emotional conflict of the parents; and (v) continued cooperation between parents to support the needs of the child.

The present study is a pilot project to shed light on the role a parental gender transposition plays in the life of the child. In a manner similar to the studies of divorce, this study is an attempt to elucidate the protective and risk factors for children with a transitioning transsexual parent. With some understanding of the complexities that underlie the effects on children of separation and divorce, these factors significantly complicate an objective evaluation regarding the role of the gender transition alone. Both sets of couples, those who choose to remain together and those who undergo separation or divorce, are necessary to tease apart the complexities of divorce from the gender transition. However, parents who choose to maintain an intact family throughout the gender transition are likely quite different from those who separate and thus, remaining as an intact family may not be protective in all situations, but only in the context of an authentic family choice.

The purpose of this study is to explore the short- and long-term adaptation of children with a transsexual parent seeking to reduce their gender dysphoria by transitioning to the opposite sex. The goal is to ascertain both risk and protective factors for children at different developmental stages at the time of the transition, and to identify the role of disclosure to the children.

METHODS

A questionnaire was developed and mailed to therapists working with transgendered clients and listed in the directory for the Harry Benjamin International Gender Dysphoria Association (HBIGDA). The form contained a number of questions in an attempt to determine the risk and protective factors for children of different genders and developmental levels. The clinicians' impressions of both the harmful and beneficial aspects of disclosure of the transition to children were also assessed for children at different developmental levels. The survey was accompanied with a cover letter that described the nature of the study and requested informed consent. No item on the survey related to any specific patient and thus the confidentiality of the individual patients who were seen by the therapists was maintained.

RESULTS

Although nearly 40 questionnaires were mailed out, only ten therapists (27%) completed and returned the forms. These therapists had an average of 14.2 years treating transgendered patients and together had seen 4,768 individuals. This was a group with considerable experience, which had likely encountered a myriad of different family constellations. However, this is a descriptive study secondary to the small number who returned the questionnaires.

Of the 4,768-transgendered individuals, the respondents reported that 2,504 (53%) transitioned to full time living in the other genetic sex. The vast majority of these individuals underwent sexual reassignment surgery (SRS). The percentage of male-to-female and female-to-male patients who were parents at the time of their transition was 64% and 47%, respectively. If a parent was planning to transition at some point, the therapists felt that non-disclosure to their children was more harmful than disclosure. However, several therapists recommended that for a parent of an adolescent, it would be best to wait until the teen had reached early adulthood, if at all possible, before both disclosing and initiating their transition.

The transition itself was rated as placing the child at mild to moderate risk; the factors that placed the child at most risk are listed in Table 1.

In rank order, those factors that place the child at most risk are: (1) an abrupt separation from either parent; (2) a spouse who is extremely opposed to the transition; (3) a personality disorder in the transitioning parent; (4) parental conflict regarding the transition; and (5) a personality disorder in the non-transitioning parent. Those factors that were rated to be most protective for the child are (also see Table 1): (1) a close emotional tie between the child and the non-transitioning parent; (2) cooperation between the parents regarding child rearing; (3) extended family supportive of the transitioning parent; (4) a close emotional relationship between the child and the transitioning parent; and (5) an ongoing contact with both parents.

The therapists were asked to rate the child's short-term reaction and long-term adaptation dependent on various developmental stages. The short-term reaction is shown in Figure 2, and the long-term adaptation is shown in Figure 1. As would be expected, family conflict considerably worsens the children's reaction in both the initial and long-term phases. Furthermore, the therapists reported that the adolescents had the most difficulty with a parent's

TABLE 1. Risk and Protective Factors for Children with a Parent Undergoing a Gender Transition

Risk Factors (in rank order from greatest risk)

- Abrupt separation from either parent
- Spouse who is extremely opposed to the transition
- Personality disorder in the transitioning parent
- Parental conflict regarding the transition
- Personality disorder in the non-transitioning parent

Protective Factors (in rank order from most protective)

- Child with close emotional ties to the non-transitioning parent
- Cooperation between parents regarding child rearing
- Extended family supportive of transitioning parent
- Child with close emotional relationship with transitioning parent
- Ongoing contact with both parents

transition, irrespective of whether it was an initial reaction or long term adaptation. It was the preschool group who are reported to do by far the best, although adults also seem to fare well with the transition, so long as there is not extensive family conflict.

CASE STUDIES

Preschooler

Katelyn, who is currently six years old, was 18 months old and an only child when her mother, Jennifer, started her transition. Growing up, Jennifer was quite the tomboy, but, due to family pressure and a strong religious upbringing, she dated, married and became pregnant in her early 20s. The body changes associated with the pregnancy were extremely difficult, and on several occasions she considered an abortion. However, due to her religious views, this was not pursued. She became depressed during her pregnancy and entered into counseling at that time. The disclosure of her difficulties to her husband during the therapy was met with confusion initially, followed by hostility, then separation.

Katelyn knows Jennifer only as Jeff, whom she calls "Pop." Her father has remarried and has primary custody; Katelyn, however, enjoys spending time at both parents' homes. She calls her step-mom, "Mom," and Jeff is supportive of this. For Christmas, she wanted to give her Pop a wallet. Katelyn has no confusion regarding her own gender identity, is happy that she is a girl, and is doing well both academically and socially.

Latency Age

Manuel is a 10-year-old male whose father, formerly Philip, now Wendy, transitioned just after Manuel turned eight. There was considerable marital conflict both prior to and after the transition. The transition started after the mother took Manuel and went to live with other family members in town. During the transition, Manuel was told by his mother that his father was "a sicko" and "a pervert" and that he shouldn't ever see him again. Manuel presented to a child and adolescent psychiatry clinic with encopresis and behavioral difficulties. Although some of the behavioral difficulties predated the transition, these were mild, and the encopresis began following the separation. Manuel has not seen his father in over two years, and the only communication between them is via a sister of the father, who spends time with Manuel and occasionally relays information to Wendy.

Adolescent

Sara is sixteen years old, the eldest of three daughters. Two years ago Sara's father, Donald, a teacher, announced his plans to have gender reassignment surgery, and to live and work full time as a female. While Sara was always closer to her father than her mother, the disclosure of her father's transgenderism was a blow. Sara had been hospitalized in the past for cutting herself, and has struggled with morbid obesity.

Today, Sara and the parent she calls Diane, are struggling to redefine their relationship. While Sara accepts her parent's gender transition, she is not anxious to talk about it. Her friends are the main focus of her life, and she is working hard to move away from her family of origin. Sara believes her parent's decision to have gender reassignment has very much complicated her own life. She has been questioning her own sexual identity for many years, and yet many see this as a by-product of her father's conflicts. While Sara claims she understands, "intellectually," why her father needed to "be Diane," she thinks it "sucks' in terms of the effect this has had on her own life.

Young Adult

Susan was 24 years old when her father abruptly told her that he had always felt female, and was planning on making a complete gender transition. Initially, Susan was confused and thought her father might be suffering from depression, or some other mental illness. She did not live at home at the time, but maintained a close relationship with both parents, who were separated. Susan sought out counseling, but the therapist had little knowledge of gender conditions. She recommended that Susan keep the communication lines open and try to educate herself as best she could about transsexualism. To that end, Susan went on the Internet and read several books.

When Susan would spend time with her father, who was now going by the name Kim, she found "Kim" to be much more pleasant and calm than "Ken" had been. This helped Susan to realize that her parent was not depressed and was honestly struggling with a little-understood, but nonetheless very genuine issue.

Today Susan and Kim have a very close and supportive relationship. Susan attributes much of the ease of their interaction to the fact that Kim is so authentically female appearing. This has made it easy for Susan to be in social situations with her parent without arousing unwanted attention or having to "explain" the situation.

DISCUSSION

The considerable experience reported by the therapists shows that children fare better overall when the transition occurs at an earlier developmental level.

The adolescent period, however, was noted to be a more difficult time for youth dealing with a parental gender transition. Since a hallmark of adolescence involves wrestling with issues of identity and roles (Erikson, 1950), it is not surprising that youth in this age group would have more difficulties with a child undergoing a gender transition. The greater difficulties with a transitioning parent during the adolescent period has been hypothesized by Green (1998b).

Green (1998b) has written about the perception that preschool children are at increased vulnerability, as this period of time corresponds with the consolidation of gender identity (formed prior to 3 years of age). Thus it is noteworthy that the therapists reported that children in the preschool years appear to make the most successful adaptation to the situation, especially in the context of minimal parental conflict.

Furthermore, neither Green's early (1978) nor later research (1998b) demonstrated any lasting interference in the consolidation of gender identity in the children he studied. Whereas adolescents would have cognitive skills to grasp the social stigma associated with transgressing gender lines, young children would not, and this may offer some protection.

None of the therapists viewed the transition itself as a neutral event, and there was a general consensus that it placed the child at mild to moderate risk.

FIGURE 1. Clinician's Risk Rating of Children According to Developmental Stage (0 = Minimal to 5 = Severe). Scores Reflect Long Term Adaptation by Children.

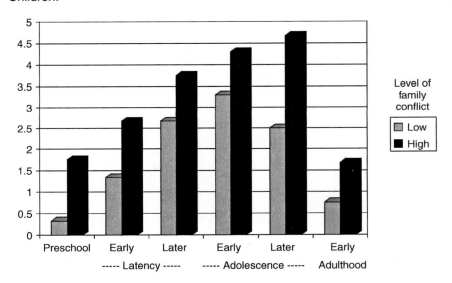

FIGURE 2. Clinician's Risk Rating of Children According to Developmental Stage (0 = Minimal to 5 = Severe). Scores Reflect Initial Reaction by the Children to the Transition.

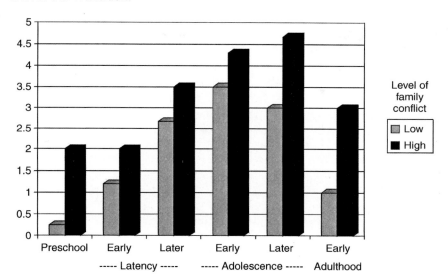

On the other hand, a ubiquitous response among therapists was that if a transsexual waited to transition until the children were older and consequently withheld all forms of disclosure, this was actually more difficult to deal with for the children. The exception is the period of later adolescence, where several therapists recommended that the parent wait, if possible, until the children had reached young adulthood. Withholding information about the potential for a parent to undergo a gender transition appears to be similar to other areas of withholding information (i.e., a child's adoption, in-vitro fertilization, etc.). If the child will likely learn, then adaptation is best when they learn early in life.

There was an overall consensus among the therapists that factors within the parental relationship and family constellation had significantly more bearing on the outcome of the children than the transition itself. Such factors as abrupt separation from the transitioning parent, non-supportive family members, parental conflict, and an inability for families to work together were all considered to place the child at risk for adjustment difficulties (Table 1). Parental conflict also adversely effected both immediate and long-term adjustment for the child (Figure 2). It is not uncommon for children to experience adversity as a result of parental illness, accidents, poverty, or marital discord. Some children, however, are able to adapt to these situations so that their development is not impeded. Researchers have studied the ability of children to spring back and recover following stressful events and designated these children as having traits of resilience (Garmezy, 1991). Some factors that are associated with resilience are intrinsic, such as temperament and personality. However, environmental influences can also contribute to fostering resilience in children (Werner, 1990).

Factors that have been shown to be associated with a resilient adaptation by children include: (i) the presence of responsive, accepting and warm parents who are concerned for the well-being of their children; (ii) supportive relationships with caring adults (i.e., a grandparent, neighbor, or teacher); (iii) role models of the same sex; (iv) positive school environment that allows students both structure and positions of responsibility; (v) teachers who are responsive and who serve as role models; (vi) social support network; (vii) and the ability of the children to demonstrate mastery in skills outside the home (i.e., sports, music, school work, work, etc.) (Bradley et al., 1994; Garmezy, 1991; Masten, Best, and Garmezy, 1990; Werner, 1989; Werner, 1990).

Research in factors associated with resilience meshes well with the reports by the therapists regarding risks and protective factors for children whose parents are undergoing a gender transition. The situation considered most protective was a child with close emotional ties to the non-transitioning parent. Parents who are able to work together can provide a more structured and nurturing environment and be more responsive to the child. Those factors that promote health of both parents, but especially the primary parent, can only benefit the children. The therapists also commented on the protective role of extended family members who are supportive of the transitioning parent. It is likely that non-supportive family members would likely increase the interfamilial conflict and potentially sabotage the relationship between the child and the transitioning parent. Finally, the therapists reported that an ongoing relationship and a close emotional tie with the transitioning parent are protective. This is supported by Green's work (1998b), who found no adverse outcomes for the children followed in his study.

There are a number of weaknesses of the present pilot study. Since the study queries therapists themselves rather than directly studying the children and adolescents, both reporting errors and sampling bias are possible. Furthermore, the number of respondents to the survey was small, although there was considerable experience among those who did respond. Studies in the future should have a prospective design and evaluate the children directly within their family constellation. Additionally, it would be helpful to know the relationship between the sex of the child and the transitioning parent (i.e., if the parent transitions to the same sex as the child, is that different than if the parent transitions to the opposite sex of the child?). In spite of the study's weaknesses, the paucity of research in this area makes this study a contribution to the existing literature.

RECOMMENDATIONS FOR THERAPISTS

Perhaps the most intuitive approach for therapists working with either parent is to promote a collaborative relationship between the parents. This will not only benefit the children, but also will very likely promote the mental health of both parents. This is not a trivial task. Green (1998a) describes a common sequence of events in which the resistance of the non-transitioning parent toward the transsexual parent's transition, often catalyzed by new relationships, family members, or health professionals, gradually erodes the transitioning parent's relationship with the children.

It is a frequent concern of the non-transitioning parent that the transition will be more harmful to the child than loss of contact with the parent. What then ensues are both overt and covert messages to the children regarding the transitioning parent, which can adversely affect the relationship. Furthermore, the transitioning parent may have feelings of being unworthy as a parent, and thus part of this withdrawal may be derived from the transitioning parent. The result is what Green (1998a) describes as a "Parental Alienation Syndrome" in which the lack of contact with the transitioning parent, coupled with the hostile response of the child's support system toward the transitioning parent, gradually alienates the parent from the child's life.

The constellation of an unsupportive former spouse and family conflict provides a challenge for the therapist working with a transitioning parent. If the patient does express feelings of unworthiness as a parent, these issues can be addressed. In spite of the conflicted relationship, it is in the best interest of the children that the custodial parent be as emotionally healthy and receptive to the children's needs as possible. The primary protective factor listed by the therapists and supported by research on protective factors for children, was a close emotional tie to the non-transitioning parent. The challenge is to work with the transitioning parent to assist them to maintain a parental role without engaging in harmful retaliatory behavior directed at the non-transitioning parent.

When the custodial parent attempts to turn the children against the transitioning parent, it can be very difficult for the latter to avoid engaging in retaliatory behavior against the former. Doing so can potentially escalate the conflict and undermine the protective relationship between the non-transitioning parent and the children. In such cases, a therapist may be tempted to foster a passive stance–such as facilitating the yielding of their parental rights–by the transitioning parent. However, since a close emotional tie with the transitioning parent is also considered a protective factor, working with the patient to obtain parental rights can be beneficial for the children.

For the therapist who is working with the non-transitioning parent who is opposed to the transition, psychoeducation will assist both the patient and those extended family members who are willing to take part. Many misperceptions exist regarding GID (i.e., that the transitioning parent could "get over it" if they tried hard enough), and education can be beneficial in some cases. The therapy goals are similar to those of the transitioning parent, namely, to reduce the level of familial conflict, support the parental roles, and to foster the development of protective factors for the child. This may include having the child involved with extended family, extracurricular activities, or consciously choosing a school that will foster the child's growth. Discussions of what to call the transitioning parent can be accomplished in the context of therapy and may include the children, especially since the use of "Mom" or "Dad" is typically reserved for the non-transitioning parent.

The therapist can work with families to help them determine what name the children will call their transitioning parent. Families can be encouraged to experiment with different names to determine what seems best for them. Some children continue to call their father "Dad," while some call her "Mom." Some will only call her "Dad" in private and use a different name when around others. Oftentimes children will refer to the transitioning parent by their first name or using "Aunt" or "Uncle." Finally, some will make up a new name just for that parent. It is a ubiquitous phenomenon that parent and child alike are uncomfortable in public with the gender term associated with their genetic sex (i.e., Mom or Dad). Furthermore, younger children seem to adapt most easily to whatever name is chosen.

Issues of grief arise in both the parents and the children, and these can be addressed during therapy. Extra support may be needed for adolescents and, if possible, a group with others in the same situation may be beneficial. Although some teens can be quite accepting ("Wow, I wish your dad was my mom!"), such a response is likely an outlier and questions regarding what teens disclose to their friends can be an issue. Helping the teenager not personalize the transition and take a more "matter-of-fact" approach can be beneficial.

CONCLUSIONS

In summary, a parental gender transition is not a neutral event in the lives of children. However, the majority of therapists reported that postponing the transition and not disclosing placed the children (except for adolescents) at greater risk than the transition itself. Factors that prove protective for children include the children being at an earlier age at the time of the gender transition, minimum familial conflict, family members working together for the welfare of their children, maintenance of contact with both the transitioning and non-transitioning parent, cooperation regarding parenting, and the extended family taking an active role in the lives of the children.

REFERENCES

Allen, M. & Burrell, N. (1996), Comparing the impact of homosexual and heterosexual parents on children: Meta-analysis of existing research. *J. Homosex.* 32:19-35.

American Academy of Pediatrics (1996), *The Classification of Child and Adolescent Mental Diagnosis in Primary Care: Diagnostic and Statistical Manual for Primary Care (DSM-PC) Child and Adolescent Version.* Elk Grove Village, Illinois: American Academy of Pediatrics.

American Psychiatric Association (1994), *Diagnostic and Statistical Manual of Mental Disorders, Fourth Edition (DSM-IV).* Washington, DC: American Psychiatric Association.

Bradley, R., Whiteside, L., Mundfrom, D., Casey, P., Kelleher, K. & Pope, S. (1994), Early indications of resilience and their relation to experiences in the home environments of low birthweight, premature children living in poverty. *Child. Dev.*, 65: 346-360.

Brewaeys, A. & van-Hall, E.V. (1997), Lesbian motherhood: The impact on child development and family functioning. *J. Psychosom. Obstet. Gynaecol.*, 18:1-16.

Crawford, I. & Solliday, E. (1996), The attitudes of undergraduate college students toward gay parenting. *J. Homosex.*, 30:63-77.

Erikson, E.H. (1950), *Childhood and Society.* New York: Norton.

Fahrner, E., Kockott, G. & Duran, G. (1987), Die Psychosoziale Integration operierter Transsexuaeller. *Nervenartzt*, 58:340-348.

Garmezy, N. (1991), Resilience in children's adaptation to negative life events and stressed environments. *Pediatrics Annual*, 20:459-466.

Gold, M.A., Perrin, E.C. & Futterman, D. (1994), Children of gay and lesbian parents. *Pediatr. Rev.* 15:354-358.

Golombok, S., Tasker, F. & Murray, C. (1997), Children raised in fatherless families from infancy: Family relationships and the socioemotional development of children of lesbian and single heterosexual mothers. *J. Child Psychol. Psychiat.*, 38:783-791.

Green, R. (1978), Sexual identity of 37 children raised by homosexual or transsexual parents. *Amer. J. Psychiat.*, 135:692-697.

_____ (1998a), Presentation at the Third International Congress on Sex and Gender, Exeter College, Oxford University.

_____ (1998b), Transsexual's children. *Int. J. Transgender*, 2:http://www.symposion.com/ijt/ijtc0601.htm.

_____ & Blanchard, R. (2000), Gender identity disorders. In: *Kaplan & Sadock's Comprehensive Textbook of Psychiatry, Vol. 1, Seventh Edition,* eds. B.J. Sadock & V.A. Sadock. Philadelphia: Lippincott, Williams & Wilkins, pp. 1646-1662.

_____, Mandel, J.B., Hotvedt, M.E., Gray, J. & Smith, L. (1986), Lesbian mothers and their children: A comparison with solo parent heterosexual mothers and their children. *Arch. Sex. Behav.*, 15:167-184.

Hetherington, E.M., Cox, M. & Cox, R. (1982), Effects of divorce on parents and children. In: *Nontraditional Families: Parenting and Child Development*, ed. M. Lamb. Hillsdale, NJ: Erlbaum, pp. 233-288.

Kalter, N., Reimer, B. & Brickman, A. (1985), Implications of divorce for female development. *J. Am. Acad. Child Psychiat.*, 24:538-544.

Keller, A.C., Althof, S.E. & Lothstein, L.M. (1982), Group therapy with gender-identity patients–a four year study. *Amer. J. Psychother.*, 36:223-228.

Kleber, D.J., Howell, R.J. & Tibbits-Kleber, A.L. (1986), The impact of parental homosexuality in child custody cases: A review of the literature. *Bull. Amer. Acad. Psychiat. Law.*,14:81-87.

Maney, D.W. & Cain, R.E. (1997), Preservice elementary teacher's attitudes toward gay and lesbian parenting. *J. Sch. Health.*, 67:236-241.

Masten, A., Best, K. & Garmezy, N. (1990), Resilience and development. *Dev. Psychopath.*, 2:425-444.

Patterson, C.J. (1992), Children of lesbian and gay parents. *Child Dev.*, 63:1025-1042.

Pauly, I.B. (1981), Outcome of sex reassignment surgery for transsexuals. *Aust. New Zeal. J. Psychol.*, 15:45-51.

Rakic, Z., Starcevic, V., Maric, J. & Kelin, K. (1996), The outcome of sex reassignment surgery in Belgrade: 32 patients of both sexes. *Arch. Sex. Behav.*, 25:515-525.

Sales, J. (1995), Children of a transsexual father: A successful intervention. *Eur. J.Child Adol. Psychiat.*, 4:136-139.

Santrock, J.W. & Warshak, R.A. (1979), Father custody and social development in boys and girls. *J. Soc. Issues*, 35:112-125.

Tasker, F. & Golombok, S. (1995), Adults raised as children in lesbian families. *Amer. J. Orthopsychiatry*, 65:203-215.

Tsoi, W.F. (1993), Follow-up study of transsexuals after sex-reassignment surgery. *Singapore Med. J.*, 34:515-517.

van-Kesteren, P.J., Gooren, L.J. & Megens, J.A. (1996), An epidemiological and demographic study of transsexuals in the Netherlands. *Arch. Sex. Behav.*, 25:589-600.

van-Nijnatten, C.H. (1995), Sexual orientation of parents and Dutch family law. *Med. Law*, 14:359-368.

Wallerstein, J.S. & Kelly J.B. (1980), *Surviving the Breakup: How Children and Their Parents Cope with Divorce*. New York, Basic Books.

_____ & Blakeslee, S. (1989), *Second Chances: Men, Women and Children a Decade After Divorce*. New York: Ticknor and Fields.

_____ & Corbin, S.B. (1989), Daughters of divorce: Report from a ten-year study. *Am. J. Orthopsychiatry*, 59:593-604.

_____ & _____ (1996), The child and the vicissitudes of divorce. In: *Child and Adolescent Psychiatry: A Comprehensive Textbook*, ed. M. Lewis. Baltimore: Williams & Wilkins, pp. 1118-1127.

Weitze, C. & Osburg, S. (1996), Transsexualism in Germany: Empirical data on epidemiology and application of the German Transsexuals' Act during its first ten years. *Arch. Sex. Behav.*, 25:409-425.

Werner, E.E. (1989), High-risk children in young adulthood: A longitudinal study from birth to 32 years. *Amer. J. Orthopsychiatry*, 52:72-81.

_____ (1990), Protective factors and individual resilience. In: *Handbook of Early Childhood Intervention*, eds. S. Meisels & J. Shonkoff. Cambridge, England: Cambridge University Press, pp. 97-116.

Zaslow, M.J. (1988), Sex differences in children's response to parental divorce. *Amer. J. Orthopsychiatry*, 58:355-378.

_____ (1989), Sex differences in children's response to parental divorce. *Amer. J. Orthopsychiatry*, 59:118-141.

Harry Benjamin and Psychiatrists

Charles L. Ihlenfeld, MD

SUMMARY. Harry Benjamin, MD, was a pioneer physician who founded the transgender field and coined the term "transsexual." Benjamin drew criticism from some in the psychiatric community when he began treating transgendered people with cross-gender hormones and encouragement in their efforts in transitioning. By and large, psychiatrists of this time considered gender dysphoria as a manifestation of significant psychopathology and considered the treatment Benjamin was then prescribing as psychiatrically contraindicated. Rather than discouraging Benjamin, this response simply reinforced his feeling that psychiatry as a discipline lacked "common sense."

The author worked with Dr. Benjamin for 6 years, was to become his heir apparent, but then left the practice to undertake a psychiatric residency. This paper chronicles changes in the author's own life and conceptual thinking about transsexualism during this time. Some years later the author finally learned the true extent of Dr. Benjamin's feelings about these events. *[Article copies available for a fee from The Haworth Document Delivery Service: 1-800-HAWORTH. E-mail address: <docdelivery@ haworthpress.com> Website: <http://www.HaworthPress.com> © 2004 by The Haworth Press, Inc. All rights reserved.]*

KEYWORDS. Harry Benjamin, homosexuality, psychiatry, psychoanalysis, sexual reassignment, transgender, transsexuality

---

Charles L. Ihlenfeld is retired from private psychiatric practice and resides on Long Island.

Address correspondence to: Charles L. Ihlenfeld, MD, P.O. Box 576, Shelter Island Heights, NY 11965-0576 (E-mail: clihlen@optonline.net).

The author wishes to thank Andrew E. Behrendt, PhD, for his invaluable suggestions and editorial assistance and William S. Packard, MD, for his constant support and encouragement.

[Haworth co-indexing entry note]: "Harry Benjamin and Psychiatrists." Ihlenfeld, Charles L. Co-published simultaneously in *Journal of Gay & Lesbian Psychotherapy* (The Haworth Medical Press, an imprint of The Haworth Press, Inc.) Vol. 8, No. 1/2, 2004, pp. 147-152; and: *Transgender Subjectivities: A Clinician's Guide* (ed: Ubaldo Leli, and Jack Drescher) The Haworth Medical Press, an imprint of The Haworth Press, Inc., 2004, pp. 147-152. Single or multiple copies of this article are available for a fee from The Haworth Document Delivery Service [1-800-HAWORTH, 9:00 a.m. - 5:00 p.m. (EST). E-mail address: docdelivery@haworthpress.com].

Digital Object Identifer: 10.1300/J236v08n01_11

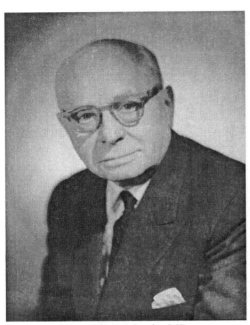

Harry S. Benjamin, MD
(1885-1986)

Fifty years after Christine Jorgensen had her surgery in Denmark, transsexualism has its own *DSM-IV* coding and gender studies is a recognized academic discipline. This was not always so. When Harry Benjamin first started treating transsexual patients with hormones he knew that he was doing something that most physicians would not do. He was aware that psychiatrists generally believed that these patients were delusional in their belief that they were in fact members of the opposite sex. Benjamin, with his anti-analytic bias and his belief that psychoanalysis was unscientific (Person, 1999), simply felt that he was right and mainstream psychiatry was wrong. I have a story of my own that suggests to me that he probably maintained this opinion to the end of his days.

Harry Benjamin never did like psychiatrists much. To be sure, he did have individual psychiatrists whom he respected and counted as friends and colleagues. As a group, however, they were not among his favorite people. His antipathy was well founded. In the 1950s and 1960s, the general psychiatric belief was that men who thought that they were women and vice versa were clearly delusional. Schizophrenia was the diagnosis of choice. Patients told him of being treated harshly by psychiatrists and other physicians with whom they had consulted. Simply put, most doctors wanted nothing to do with these patients, and some were more emphatic in declaring this than others. As a result, many patients were reluctant to subject themselves to further abuse by making additional efforts to find help. And if doctors thought that these patients were crazy, one can only imagine what they thought of a fellow physician who suggested that just maybe these patients had a point that most doctors were missing. He met this skepticism personally when he gave talks at hospitals and professional meetings and heard the questions and often-critical comments from psychiatrists in attendance.

Harry Benjamin received his medical degree from the University of Tübingen in Germany in 1912. He first came to the United States in 1913 to do work with a promising new treatment for tuberculosis. When he tried to return to Germany in 1914, his ship missed clearing English waters by half an hour and was diverted to England at the outbreak of World War I. Several months later he came back to New York City and established his own private, general medical practice (Person, 1999, pp. 354-355). In the decades that followed, he pursued his interests in the developing fields of endocrinology, gerontology, and sexology and was among the first to try hormonal and surgical treatments for aging.

Thus, when in the 1930s one of his older patients, a cross-dressing man, asked him for female hormones, Harry Benjamin had a good idea of what the physical effects would be. He knew this patient quite well, and realized that the man was not crazy. The man himself knew his physician well enough to feel safe in making the request and, in fact, responded well to the treatment. He felt calmer, happier, and more content and showed no ill effects from the hormones.

This story shows us the genius of Harry Benjamin: he was willing to listen to his patients without prejudice and to learn from his work with them.

I met Harry Benjamin on April Fool's Day of 1969. A friend who had arranged the introduction told me that Benjamin needed someone to cover his office for the coming summer. As a young internist with an interest in endocrinology, I seemed a likely prospect for a practice that largely involved hormonal treatment of transsexual patients. My friend gently advised me not to get too involved.

Harry Benjamin was then 84 years old. Through his pioneering work in the field, he had made transsexualism a recognized medical term. In 1966 he had written *The Transsexual Phenomenon* (Benjamin, 1966), at the time the only book on the subject written for a medical audience. I was impressed by this distinguished figure sitting behind his desk, speaking quietly with a soft German accent. He was warm, friendly, and very clear about what he was doing with his patients. A few short weeks later, he flew to San Francisco and left me as the resident expert in his office. In the time-honored tradition of "see-one-do-one-teach-one," I learned on the job. It was not until much later that I realized that Harry Benjamin had learned about these patients and their concerns in exactly the same way that he had let me learn about them.

As I got to know Harry Benjamin, I learned something else about him: he knew who his friends were. He had spent too much time working outside mainstream medicine not to realize that physicians as a lot tended to be conservative. They wanted to offend neither their patients nor their peers. Hospitals and universities were sensitive to the opinions of their major donors. He thought of himself as a persistent pioneer. His willingness to work with new and sometimes controversial treatments, in fields such as sex and aging, meant that often he had to work alone. He valued those colleagues who understood and supported what he was doing. Their friendship and personal loyalty to him were profoundly important.

Fast-forward to 1975: a lot had changed for Harry Benjamin. The summer of 1975 was his last in San Francisco. While there, he developed facial herpes. He was hospitalized for a few days with what was probably a mild encephalitis. He returned to New York City in September, never to leave again. He lived out his days at home with Gretchen, his bride of over 60 years, whom he had married when he was 40. They had no children. He died in August of 1986 at the age of 101. His heart gave out before his mind.

A lot had changed for me, too. I did not take my friend's advice. Indeed, I became deeply involved with Harry and his work. I came to appreciate the difference between *gender identity*–how one sees oneself in terms of gender–and *sexual orientation*–the role that gender preference plays in one's choice of a sexual partner. I came to know that there are infinite variations and combinations of masculinity and femininity within each of us. I was awed by the courage of people who were willing to risk losing everything to gain the truth of their own lives. Finally, at the age of 35, I understood that I was and always had been gay. I wanted to be as honest in my life as my patients were in theirs. In 1973 I came out. Harry was surprised, but very supportive when I told him.

Then I faced another change: ever more aware of the psychologic dimensions of human sexuality, I knew that I did not want to spend the rest of my career working as an amateur psychiatrist. So, in 1975 I left Harry's practice and began my psychiatric residency. This did not make Harry happy. I had been his successor, entrusted with his legacy. Now I seemed to be joining the enemy. At 90, he saw the practice he had nurtured for so many years disappearing. I am sure he felt betrayed. Our personal relationship, however, seemed to me to continue essentially unchanged.

In the fall of 1976, I was in a residency program that had a strong analytic tradition. Many of the teachers and supervisors were trained as analysts. Long-term individual psychotherapy was still a cornerstone of the program. All of this was good. However, the program's attitude about homosexuality was subtle but clear: when I told the Director of Residency Training that I was gay, he looked a little puzzled and replied, "You mean there are gay psychiatrists?"

I had a call from Daniel Greene, a writer for *The National Observer*. He was doing an article about transsexuals and asked to interview me. I met him for a long lunch on Columbus Avenue in Manhattan one weekday afternoon. We spoke first about the field in general, and then about my decision to leave Harry's practice and become a psychiatrist. I told him how I met Harry Benjamin, how working with our patients had helped me come to terms with my own sexuality, how I felt the need to understand more about my patients and the work we were doing together. Speaking as a second year resident in psychiatry, I suggested that I might have been confusing some of my own needs for acceptance and understanding with my transsexual patients' needs for understanding and liberation. In my early years in the field, I had written and spoken about the idea that transsexuals were somehow simply born with the body of one sex and the mind of the other. I told my interviewer that I no longer considered this an adequate and satisfactory explanation for what our patients experienced. I was concerned that there were psychologic issues that hormones and surgery did not reach. I feared that these unexplored and unresolved issues might resurface in later years and leave our patients with a vague but lingering sense of dissatisfaction with their lives. In a sidebar headlined about my thoughts he closed with this quotation: "Whatever surgery did, it did not fulfill a basic yearning for something that is difficult to define. This goes along with the idea that we are trying to treat something that is much deeper. It may also mean that if you are born to be a transsexual, you are doomed never to be totally happy" (Greene, 1976).

Harry and I never discussed the article.

In 1979, Janice Raymond quoted from this article in her book *The Transsexual Empire* (Raymond, 1979). She says, "*The Transsexual Empire* is basically the medical conglomerate that has created the treatment and technology that makes anatomical sex conversion possible" (pp. xiv-xv). She describes my leaving the field as "a significant defection from the transsexual empire" (p. 212). Controversial and widely read, this book brought my interview to many who had not seen the original article and insured that my words would not soon be forgotten. Less than a year ago, I had an e-mail message from a former patient who had only recently read of my comments in the *National Observer* article and wondered about my apparent decision not to support sex reassignment surgery. I assume that she saw my comments in Raymond's book.

Fast-forward to the present: I still have not taken my friend's advice. I moved to eastern Long Island in the mid-1980s and opened my own psychiatric practice. I continued to see transsexual patients both for evaluation and for counseling. I continue to this day to support hormonal and surgical reassignment when that seems appropriate. For a long time now I have known that Harry and I never disagreed on the important points. He knew from his own clinical experience that for certain patients transitioning with hormones and surgery is not only helpful, but often necessary as the only treatment we have to offer. I believe that whatever the causes–genetic, biologic, psychologic– cross gender feelings strong enough to bring a person to reassignment are probably fixed in personality far too early and far too firmly to reconcile any other way. Reassignment is simply too difficult to undertake for any lesser reason. I have had the privilege of knowing some patients for 30 years. I know that these feelings do not go away with time, and I know that through reassignment many patients have found happiness and a personal fulfillment that simply would not have been possible otherwise.

Postscript: About a year ago, when I was closing my practice, I found a letter written in longhand by Harry in May of 1978 (Benjamin, 1978). In this addendum to his will, he directs his attorney to replace me as a trustee (of what I no longer know) with an old friend. He wrote, "Dr. Ihlenfeld whom I appreciate and value as a friend, has changed psychologically thru–to my mind–the destructive influence of today's psychoanalysis which–again to my mind–replaces too often common sense by a lot of dogmatic non-sense."

He was then 93 years old. He never did like psychiatrists much.

REFERENCES

Benjamin, H. (1966), *The Transsexual Phenomenon*. New York: Julian Press.
_____ (1978), Personal communication.
Greene, D. (1976), A doctor tells why he'll no longer treat transsexuals. *The National Observer*, October 16, 1976, p. 14.
Person, E. S. (1999), Harry Benjamin and the birth of a shared cultural fantasy. In: *The Sexual Century*. New Haven, CT: Yale University Press, pp. 347-366.
Raymond, J.G. (1979), *The Transsexual Empire: The Making of the She-Male*. Boston, MA: Beacon Press.

Pronouns

Irene Willis

When my son first told me, I didn't realize
I'd have to change the pronouns,
shift their shapes to those I couldn't
fit my mouth around, or swallow.
He him his rolled off my tongue like
marbles into the box of *she her hers.*
Where were the antecedents? *Whose?*
I whirled, searching our family of names.
Who was closest? Whom to blame?
But blame implies misdeed, and here was none.
My son, *mine.* I'd never had a daughter, never knew
I would give birth in what is now called "young old age."
Mother. Father. I grasped each noun like the pole
of a carousel. When I got off
the ground was moving still, and I was holding
his gold-embroidered past, and mine.

Irene Willis's poems have appeared in *Crazyhorse, Florida Review, Laurel Review, Literary Review, New York Quarterly,* and other publications. Her first collection of poems was entitled *They Tell Me You Danced* (University Press of Florida), and she is at work on her second. She was recently awarded a residency at the Millay Colony for the Arts.

Address correspondence to: Irene Willis, 2 Cornwall Drive, Gt. Barrington, MA 01230-1592 (E-mail: irenej@vgernet.net).

[Haworth co-indexing entry note]: "Pronouns." Willis, Irene. Co-published simultaneously in *Journal of Gay & Lesbian Psychotherapy* (The Haworth Medical Press, an imprint of The Haworth Press, Inc.) Vol. 8, No. 1/2, 2004, p. 153; and: *Transgender Subjectivities: A Clinician's Guide* (ed: Ubaldo Leli, and Jack Drescher) The Haworth Medical Press, an imprint of The Haworth Press, Inc., 2004, p. 153. Single or multiple copies of this article are available for a fee from The Haworth Document Delivery Service [1-800-HAWORTH, 9:00 a.m. - 5:00 p.m. (EST). E-mail address: docdelivery@haworthpress.com].

Digital Object Identifer: 10.1300/J236v08n01_12

Index

14 stage model, 41-67. *See also* Identity formation (fourteen stage model)

BOOK ORDER FORM!

Order a copy of this book with this form or online at:
http://www.haworthpress.com/store/product.asp?sku=5282

Transgender Subjectivities
A Clinician's Guide

____ in softbound at $19.95 (ISBN: 0-7890-2576-0)
____ in hardbound at $39.95 (ISBN: 0-7890-2575-2)

COST OF BOOKS _____

POSTAGE & HANDLING _____
US: $4.00 for first book & $1.50
for each additional book
Outside US: $5.00 for first book
& $2.00 for each additional book.

SUBTOTAL _____
In Canada: add 7% GST. _____

STATE TAX _____
CA, IL, IN, MN, NY, OH & SD residents
please add appropriate local sales tax.

FINAL TOTAL _____
If paying in Canadian funds, convert
using the current exchange rate,
UNESCO coupons welcome.

❑ **BILL ME LATER:**
Bill-me option is good on US/Canada/
Mexico orders only; not good to jobbers,
wholesalers, or subscription agencies.

❑ **Signature** _____

❑ **Payment Enclosed: $** _____

❑ **PLEASE CHARGE TO MY CREDIT CARD:**
❑ Visa ❑ MasterCard ❑ AmEx ❑ Discover
❑ Diner's Club ❑ Eurocard ❑ JCB

Account # _____

Exp Date _____

Signature _____
(Prices in US dollars and subject to change without notice.)

PLEASE PRINT ALL INFORMATION OR ATTACH YOUR BUSINESS CARD
Name
Address
City   State/Province   Zip/Postal Code
Country
Tel   Fax
E-Mail

May we use your e-mail address for confirmations and other types of information? ❑ Yes ❑ No We appreciate receiving
your e-mail address. Haworth would like to e-mail special discount offers to you, as a preferred customer.
We will never share, rent, or exchange your e-mail address. We regard such actions as an invasion of your privacy.

Order From Your **Local Bookstore** or Directly From
The Haworth Press, Inc. 10 Alice Street, Binghamton, New York 13904-1580 • USA
Call Our toll-free number (1-800-429-6784) / Outside US/Canada: (607) 722-5857
Fax: 1-800-895-0582 / Outside US/Canada: (607) 771-0012
E-mail your order to us: orders@haworthpress.com

For orders outside US and Canada, you may wish to order through your local
sales representative, distributor, or bookseller.
For information, see http://haworthpress.com/distributors

(Discounts are available for individual orders in US and Canada only, not booksellers/distributors.)

Please photocopy this form for your personal use.
www.HaworthPress.com

BOF04